AIR FRYER RECIPES 2022

DELICIOUS AND EASY RECIPES FOR BEGINNERS

SARAH MELTON

Table of Contents

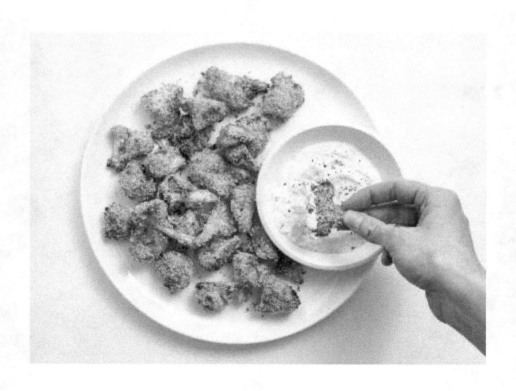

Creamy Endives

Preparation time: 10 minutes **Cooking time:** 10 minutes
Servings: 6

Ingredients:

- 6 endives, trimmed and halved
- 1 teaspoon garlic powder
- ½ cup Greek yogurt
- ½ teaspoon curry powder
- Salt and black pepper to the taste
- 3 tablespoons lemon juice

Directions:

1. In a bowl, mix endives with garlic powder, yogurt, curry powder, salt, pepper and lemon juice, toss, leave aside for 10 minutes and transfer to your preheated air fryer at 350 degrees F.
2. Cook endives for 10 minutes, divide them on plates and serve as a side dish.

Enjoy!

Nutrition: calories 100, fat 2, fiber 2, carbs 7, protein 4

Delicious Roasted Carrots

Preparation time: 10 minutes **Cooking time:** 20 minutes
Servings: 4

Ingredients:

- 1 pound baby carrots
- 2 teaspoons olive oil
- 1 teaspoon herbs de Provence
- 4 tablespoons orange juice

Directions:

1. In your air fryer's basket, mix carrots with herbs de Provence, oil and orange juice, toss and cook at 320 degrees F for 20 minutes.
2. Divide among plates and serve as a side dish.

Enjoy!

Nutrition: calories 112, fat 2, fiber 3, carbs 4, protein 3

Vermouth Mushrooms

Preparation time: 10 minutes **Cooking time:** 25 minutes
Servings: 4

Ingredients:
- 1 tablespoon olive oil
- 2 pounds white mushrooms
- 2 tablespoons white vermouth
- 2 teaspoons herbs de Provence
- 2 garlic cloves, minced

Directions:
1. In your air fryer, mix oil with mushrooms, herbs de Provence and garlic, toss and cook at 350 degrees F for 20 minutes.
2. Add vermouth, toss and cook for 5 minutes more.
3. Divide among plates and serve as a side dish.

Enjoy!

Nutrition: calories 121, fat 2, fiber 5, carbs 7, protein 4

Roasted Parsnips

Preparation time: 10 minutes **Cooking time:** 40 minutes

Servings: 6

Ingredients:

- 2 pounds parsnips, peeled and cut into medium chunks
- 2 tablespoons maple syrup
- 1 tablespoon parsley flakes, dried
- 1 tablespoon olive oil

Directions:

1. Preheat your air fryer at 360 degrees F, add oil and heat it up as well.
2. Add parsnips, parsley flakes and maple syrup, toss and cook them for 40 minutes.
3. Divide among plates and serve as a side dish.

Enjoy!

Nutrition: calories 124, fat 3, fiber 3, carbs 7, protein 4

Barley Risotto

Preparation time: 10 minutes **Cooking time:** 30 minutes

Servings: 8

Ingredients:

- 5 cups veggie stock
- 3 tablespoons olive oil
- 2 yellow onions, chopped
- 2 garlic cloves, minced
- ¾ pound barley
- 3 ounces mushrooms, sliced
- 2 ounces skim milk
- 1 teaspoon thyme, dried
- 1 teaspoon tarragon, dried
- Salt and black pepper to the taste
- 2 pounds sweet potato, peeled and chopped

Directions:

1. Put stock in a pot, add barley, stir, bring to a boil over medium heat and cook for 15 minutes.
2. Heat up your air fryer at 350 degrees F, add oil and heat it up.

3. Add barley, onions, garlic, mushrooms, milk, salt, pepper, tarragon and sweet potato, stir and cook for 15 minutes more.
4. Divide among plates and serve as a side dish.

Enjoy!

Nutrition: calories 124, fat 4, fiber 4, carbs 6, protein 4

Glazed Beets

Preparation time: 10 minutes **Cooking time:** 40 minutes

Servings: 8

Ingredients:

- 3 pounds small beets, trimmed
- 4 tablespoons maple syrup
- 1 tablespoon duck fat

Directions:

1. Heat up your air fryer at 360 degrees F, add duck fat and heat it up.
2. Add beets and maple syrup, toss and cook for 40 minutes.
3. Divide among plates and serve as a side dish.

Enjoy!

Nutrition: calories 121, fat 3, fiber 2, carbs 3, protein 4

Beer Risotto

Preparation time: 10 minutes **Cooking time:** 30 minutes

Servings: 4

Ingredients:

- 2 tablespoons olive oil
- 2 yellow onions, chopped
- 1 cup mushrooms, sliced
- 1 teaspoon basil, dried
- 1 teaspoon oregano, dried
- 1 and ½ cups rice
- 2 cups beer
- 2 cups chicken stock
- 1 tablespoon butter
- ½ cup parmesan, grated

Directions:

1. In a dish that fits your air fryer, mix oil with onions, mushrooms, basil and oregano and stir.
2. Add rice, beer, butter, stock and butter, stir again, place in your air fryer's basket and cook at 350 degrees F for 30 minutes.
3. Divide among plates and serve with grated parmesan on top as a side dish.

Enjoy!

Nutrition: calories 142, fat 4, fiber 4, carbs 6, protein 4

Cauliflower Rice

Preparation time: 10 minutes **Cooking time:** 40 minutes

Servings: 8

Ingredients:

- 1 tablespoon peanut oil
- 1 tablespoon sesame oil
- 4 tablespoons soy sauce
- 3 garlic cloves, minced
- 1 tablespoon ginger, grated
- Juice from ½ lemon
- 1 cauliflower head, riced
- 9 ounces water chestnuts, drained
- ¾ cup peas
- 15 ounces mushrooms, chopped
- 1 egg, whisked

Directions:

1. In your air fryer, mix cauliflower rice with peanut oil, sesame oil, soy sauce, garlic, ginger and lemon juice, stir, cover and cook at 350 degrees F for 20 minutes.
2. Add chestnuts, peas, mushrooms and egg, toss and cook at 360 degrees F for 20 minutes more.
3. Divide among plates and serve for breakfast.

Enjoy!

Nutrition: calories 142, fat 3, fiber 2, carbs 6, protein 4

Carrots and Rhubarb

Preparation time: 10 minutes **Cooking time:** 40 minutes
Servings: 4

Ingredients:
- 1 pound baby carrots
- 2 teaspoons walnut oil
- 1 pound rhubarb, roughly chopped
- 1 orange, peeled, cut into medium segments and zest grated
- ½ cup walnuts, halved
- ½ teaspoon stevia

Directions:

1. Put the oil in your air fryer, add carrots, toss and fry them at 380 degrees F for 20 minutes.
2. Add rhubarb, orange zest, stevia and walnuts, toss and cook for 20 minutes more.
3. Add orange segments, toss and serve as a side dish.

Enjoy!

Nutrition: calories 172, fat 2, fiber 3, carbs 4, protein 4

Roasted Eggplant

Preparation time: 10 minutes **Cooking time:** 20 minutes
Servings: 6

Ingredients:

- 1 and ½ pounds eggplant, cubed
- 1 tablespoon olive oil
- 1 teaspoon garlic powder
- 1 teaspoon onion powder
- 1 teaspoon sumac
- 2 teaspoons za'atar
- Juice from ½ lemon
- 2 bay leaves

Directions:

1. In your air fryer, mix eggplant cubes with oil, garlic powder, onion powder, sumac, za'atar, lemon juice and bay leaves, toss and cook at 370 degrees F for 20 minutes.
2. Divide among plates and serve as a side dish.

Enjoy!

Nutrition: calories 172, fat 4, fiber 7, carbs 12, protein 3

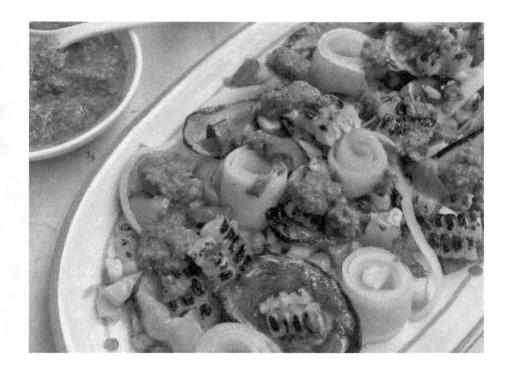

Delicious Air Fried Broccoli

Preparation time: 10 minutes **Cooking time:** 20 minutes
Servings: 4

Ingredients:

- 1 tablespoon duck fat
- 1 broccoli head, florets separated
- 3 garlic cloves, minced
- Juice from ½ lemon
- 1 tablespoon sesame seeds

Directions:

1. Heat up your air fryer at 350 degrees F, add duck fat and heat as well.
2. Add broccoli, garlic, lemon juice and sesame seeds, toss and cook for 20 minutes.
3. Divide among plates and serve as a side dish.

Enjoy!

Nutrition: calories 132, fat 3, fiber 3, carbs 6, protein 4

Onion Rings Side Dish

Preparation time: 10 minutes **Cooking time:** 10 minutes

Servings: 3

Ingredients:

- 1 onion cut into medium slices and rings separated
- 1 and ¼ cups white flour
- A pinch of salt
- 1 egg
- 1 cup milk
- 1 teaspoon baking powder
- ¾ cup bread crumbs

Directions:

1. In a bowl, mix flour with salt and baking powder, stir, dredge onion rings in this mix and place them on a separate plate.
2. Add milk and egg to flour mix and whisk well.
3. Dip onion rings in this mix, dredge them in breadcrumbs, put them in your air fryer's basket and cook them at 360 degrees F for 10 minutes.
4. Divide among plates and serve as a side dish for a steak.

Enjoy!

Nutrition: calories 140, fat 8, fiber 20, carbs 12, protein 3

Rice and Sausage Side Dish

Preparation time: 10 minutes **Cooking time:** 20 minutes
Servings: 4

Ingredients:

- 2 cups white rice, already boiled
- 1 tablespoon butter
- Salt and black pepper to the taste
- 4 garlic cloves, minced
- 1 pork sausage, chopped
- 2 tablespoons carrot, chopped
- 3 tablespoons cheddar cheese, grated
- 2 tablespoons mozzarella cheese, shredded

Directions:

1. Heat up your air fryer at 350 degrees F, add butter, melt it, add garlic, stir and brown for 2 minutes.
2. Add sausage, salt, pepper, carrots and rice, stir and cook at 350 degrees F for 10 minutes.
3. Add cheddar and mozzarella, toss, divide among plates and serve as a side dish.

Enjoy!

Nutrition: calories 240, fat 12, fiber 5, carbs 20, protein 13

Potatoes Patties

Preparation time: 10 minutes **Cooking time:** 8 minutes
Servings: 4

Ingredients:

- 4 potatoes, cubed, boiled and mashed
- 1 cup parmesan, grated
- Salt and black pepper to the taste
- A pinch of nutmeg
- 2 egg yolks
- 2 tablespoons white flour
- 3 tablespoons chives, chopped

For the breading:

- ¼ cup white flour
- 3 tablespoons vegetable oil
- 2 eggs, whisked
- ¼ cup bread crumbs

Directions:

1. In a bowl, mix mashed potatoes with egg yolks, salt, pepper, nutmeg, parmesan, chives and 2 tablespoons

flour, stir well, shape medium cakes and place them on a plate.

2. In another bowl, mix vegetable oil with bread crumbs and stir,.

3. Put whisked eggs in a third bowl and ¼ cup flour in a forth one.

4. Dip cakes in flour, then in eggs and in breadcrumbs at the end, place them in your air fryer's basket, cook them at 390 degrees F for 8 minutes, divide among plates and serve as a side dish.

Enjoy!

Nutrition: calories 140, fat 3, fiber 4, carbs 17, protein 4

Simple Potato Chips

Preparation time: 30 minutes **Cooking time:** 30 minutes
Servings: 4

Ingredients:
- 4 potatoes, scrubbed, peeled into thin chips, soaked in water for 30 minutes, drained and pat dried
- Salt the taste
- 1 tablespoon olive oil
- 2 teaspoons rosemary, chopped

Directions:
1. In a bowl, mix potato chips with salt and oil toss to coat, place them in your air fryer's basket and cook at 330 degrees F for 30 minutes.
2. Divide among plates, sprinkle rosemary all over and serve as a side dish.

Enjoy!

Nutrition: calories 200, fat 4, fiber 4, carbs 14, protein 5

Avocado Fries

Preparation time: 10 minutes **Cooking time:** 10 minutes
Servings: 4

Ingredients:

- 1 avocado, pitted, peeled, sliced and cut into medium fries
- Salt and black pepper to the taste
- ½ cup panko bread crumbs
- 1 tablespoon lemon juice
- 1 egg, whisked
- 1 tablespoon olive oil

Directions:

1. In a bowl, mix panko with salt and pepper and stir.

2. In another bowl, mix egg with a pinch of salt and whisk.

3. In a third bowl, mix avocado fries with lemon juice and oil and toss.

4. Dip fries in egg, then in panko, place them in your air fryer's basket and cook at 390 degrees F for 10 minutes, shaking halfway.

5. Divide among plates and serve as a side dish.

Enjoy!

Nutrition: calories 130, fat 11, fiber 3, carbs 16, protein 4

Veggie Fries

Preparation time: 10 minutes **Cooking time:** 30 minutes
Servings: 4

Ingredients:

- 4 parsnips, cut into medium sticks
- 2 sweet potatoes cut into medium sticks
- 4 mixed carrots cut into medium sticks
- Salt and black pepper to the taste
- 2 tablespoons rosemary, chopped
- 2 tablespoons olive oil
- 1 tablespoon flour
- ½ teaspoon garlic powder

Directions:

1. Put veggie fries in a bowl, add oil, garlic powder, salt, pepper, flour and rosemary and toss to coat.
2. Put sweet potatoes in your preheated air fryer, cook them for 10 minutes at 350 degrees F and transfer them to a platter.
3. Put parsnip fries in your air fryer, cook for 5 minutes and transfer over potato fries.

4. Put carrot fries in your air fryer, cook for 15 minutes at 350 degrees F and transfer to the platter with the other fries.
5. Divide veggie fries on plates and serve them as a side dish.

Enjoy!

Nutrition: calories 100, fat 0, fiber 4, carbs 7, protein 4

Air Fried Creamy Cabbage

Preparation time: 10 minutes **Cooking time:** 20 minute

Servings: 4

Ingredients:

- 1 green cabbage head, chopped
- 1 yellow onion, chopped
- Salt and black pepper to the taste
- 4 bacon slices, chopped
- 1 cup whipped cream
- 2 tablespoons cornstarch

Directions:

1. Put cabbage, bacon and onion in your air fryer.
2. In a bowl, mix cornstarch with cream, salt and pepper, stir and add over cabbage.
3. Toss, cook at 400 degrees F for 20 minutes, divide among plates and serve as a side dish.

Enjoy!

Nutrition: calories 208, fat 10, fiber 3, carbs 16, protein 5

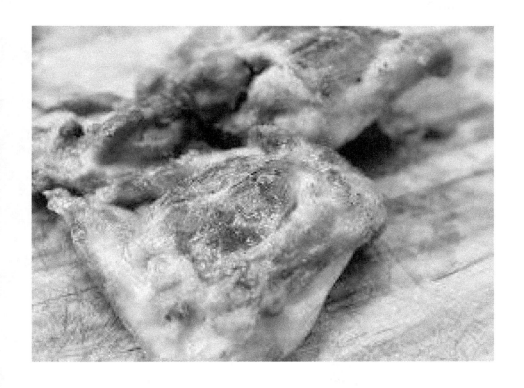

Tortilla Chips

Preparation time: 10 minutes **Cooking time:** 6 minutes
Servings: 4

Ingredients:

- 8 corn tortillas, cut into triangles
- Salt and black pepper to the taste
- 1 tablespoon olive oil
- A pinch of garlic powder
- A pinch of sweet paprika

Directions:

1. In a bowl, mix tortilla chips with oil, add salt, pepper, garlic powder and paprika, toss well, place them in your air fryer's basket and cook them at 400 degrees F for 6 minutes.
2. Serve them as a side for a fish dish.

Enjoy!

Nutrition: calories 53, fat 1, fiber 1, carbs 6, protein 4

Zucchini Croquettes

Preparation time: 10 minutes **Cooking time:** 10 minutes
Servings: 4

Ingredients:

- 1 carrot, grated
- 1 zucchini, grated
- 2 slices of bread, crumbled
- 1 egg
- Salt and black pepper to the taste
- ½ teaspoon sweet paprika
- 1 teaspoon garlic, minced
- 2 tablespoons parmesan cheese, grated
- 1 tablespoon corn flour

Directions:

1. Put zucchini in a bowl, add salt, leave aside for 10 minutes, squeeze excess water and transfer them to another bowl.
2. Add carrots, salt, pepper, paprika, garlic, flour, parmesan, egg and bread crumbs, stir well, shape 8

croquettes, place them in your air fryer and cook at 360 degrees F for 10 minutes.

3. Divide among plates and serve as a side dish

Enjoy!

Nutrition: calories 100, fat 3, fiber 1, carbs 7, protein 4

Creamy Potatoes

Preparation time: 10 minutes **Cooking time:** 20 minutes

Servings: 4

Ingredients:

- 1 an ½ pounds potatoes, peeled and cubed
- 2 tablespoons olive oil
- Salt and black pepper to the taste
- 1 tablespoon hot paprika
- 1 cup Greek yogurt

Directions:

1. Put potatoes in a bowl, add water to cover, leave aside for 10 minutes, drain, pat dry them, transfer to another bowl, add salt, pepper, paprika and half of the oil and toss them well.
2. Put potatoes in your air fryer's basket and cook at 360 degrees F for 20 minutes.
3. In a bowl, mix yogurt with salt, pepper and the rest of the oil and whisk.
4. Divide potatoes on plates, drizzle yogurt dressing all over, toss them and serve as a side dish.

Enjoy!

Nutrition: calories 170, fat 3, fiber 5, carbs 20, protein 5

Mushroom Cakes

Preparation time: 10 minutes **Cooking time:** 8 minutes **Servings:** 8

Ingredients:

- 4 ounces mushrooms, chopped
- 1 yellow onion, chopped
- Salt and black pepper to the taste
- ½ teaspoon nutmeg, ground
- 2 tablespoons olive oil
- 1 tablespoon butter
- 1 and ½ tablespoon flour
- 1 tablespoon bread crumbs
- 14 ounces milk

Directions:

1. Heat up a pan with the butter over medium high heat, add onion and mushrooms, stir, cook for 3 minutes, add flour, stir well again and take off heat.
2. Add milk gradually, salt, pepper and nutmeg, stir and leave aside to cool down completely.
3. In a bowl, mix oil with bread crumbs and whisk.

4. Take spoonfuls of the mushroom filling, add to breadcrumbs mix, coat well, shape patties out of this mix, place them in your air fryer's basket and cook at 400 degrees F for 8 minutes.
5. Divide among plates and serve as a side for a steak

Enjoy!

Nutrition: calories 192, fat 2, fiber 1, carbs 16, protein 6

Creamy Roasted Peppers Side Dish

Preparation time: 10 minutes **Cooking time:** 10 minutes
Servings: 4

Ingredients:

- 1 tablespoon lemon juice
- 1 red bell pepper
- 1 green bell pepper
- 1 yellow bell pepper
- 1 lettuce head, cut into strips
- 1 ounce rocket leaves
- Salt and black pepper to the taste
- 3 tablespoons Greek yogurt
- 2 tablespoons olive oil

Directions:

1. Place bell peppers in your air fryer's basket, cook at
   400 degrees F for 10 minutes, transfer to a bowl, leave
   aside for 10 minutes, peel them, discard seeds, cut

them in strips, transfer to a larger bowl, add rocket leaves and lettuce strips and toss.

2. In a bowl, mix oil with lemon juice, yogurt, salt and pepper and whisk well.

3. Add this over bell peppers mix, toss to coat, divide among plates and serve as a side salad.

Enjoy!

Nutrition: calories 170, fat 1, fiber 1, carbs 2, protein 6

Greek Veggie Side Dish

Preparation time: 10 minutes **Cooking time:** 45 minutes
Servings: 4

Ingredients:

- 1 eggplant, sliced
- 1 zucchini, sliced
- 2 red bell peppers, chopped
- 2 garlic cloves, minced
- 3 tablespoons olive oil
- 1 bay leaf
- 1 thyme spring, chopped
- 2 onions, chopped
- 4 tomatoes, cut into quarters
- Salt and black pepper to the taste

Directions:

1. In your air fryer's pan, mix eggplant slices with zucchini ones, bell peppers, garlic, oil, bay leaf, thyme, onions, tomatoes, salt and pepper, toss and cook them at 300 degrees F for 35 minutes.
2. Divide among plates and serve as a side dish.

Enjoy!

Nutrition: calories 200, fat 1, fiber 3, carbs 7, protein 6

Yellow Squash and Zucchinis Side Dish

Preparation time: 10 minutes **Cooking time:** 35 minutes

Servings: 4

Ingredients:

- 6 teaspoons olive oil
- 1 pound zucchinis, sliced
- ½ pound carrots, cubed
- 1 yellow squash, halved, deseeded and cut into chunks
- Salt and white pepper to the taste
- 1 tablespoon tarragon, chopped

Directions:

1. In your air fryer's basket, mix zucchinis with carrots, squash, salt, pepper and oil, toss well and cook at 400 degrees F for 25 minutes.
2. Divide them on plates and serve as a side dish with tarragon sprinkled on top.

Enjoy!

Nutrition: calories 160, fat 2, fiber 1, carbs 5, protein 5

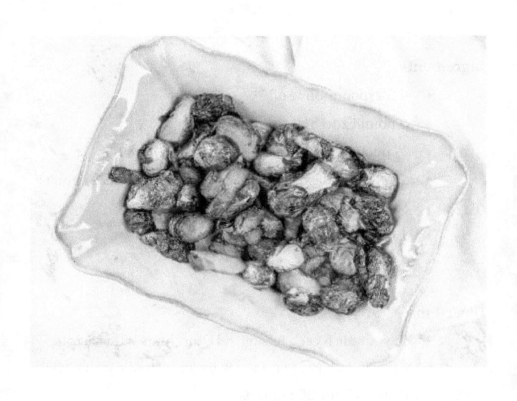

Flavored Cauliflower Side Dish

Preparation time: 10 minutes **Cooking time:** 10 minutes
Servings: 4

Ingredients:

- 12 cauliflower florets, steamed
- Salt and black pepper to the taste
- ¼ teaspoon turmeric powder
- 1 and ½ teaspoon red chili powder
- 1 tablespoon ginger, grated
- 2 teaspoons lemon juice
- 3 tablespoons white flour
- 2 tablespoons water
- Cooking spray
- ½ teaspoon corn flour

Directions:

1. In a bowl, mix chili powder with turmeric powder, ginger paste, salt, pepper, lemon juice, white flour, corn flour and water, stir, add cauliflower, toss well and transfer them to your air fryer's basket.

2. Coat them with cooking spray, cook them at 400 degrees F for 10 minutes, divide among plates and serve as a side dish.

Enjoy!

Nutrition: calories 70, fat 1, fiber 2, carbs 12, protein 3

Coconut Cream Potato es

Preparation time: 10 minutes **Cooking time:** 20 minutes
Servings: 4

Ingredients:

- 2 eggs, whisked
- Salt and black pepper to the taste
- 1 tablespoon cheddar cheese, grated
- 1 tablespoon flour
- 2 potatoes, sliced
- 4 ounces coconut cream

Directions:

1. Place potato slices in your air fryer's basket and cook at 360 degrees F for 10 minutes.
2. Meanwhile, in a bowl, mix eggs with coconut cream, salt, pepper and flour.
3. Arrange potatoes in your air fryer's pan, add coconut cream mix over them, sprinkle cheese, return to air fryer's basket and cook at 400 degrees F for 10 minutes more.
4. Divide among plates and serve as a side dish.

Enjoy!

Nutrition: calories 170, fat 4, fiber 1, carbs 15, protein 17

Cajun Onion Wedges

Preparation time: 10 minutes **Cooking time:** 15 minutes

Servings: 4

Ingredients:

- 2 big white onions, cut into wedges
- Salt and black pepper to the taste
- 2 eggs
- ¼ cup milk
- 1/3 cup panko
- A drizzle of olive oil
- 1 and ½ teaspoon paprika
- 1 teaspoon garlic powder
- ½ teaspoon Cajun seasoning

Directions:

1. In a bowl, mix panko with Cajun seasoning and oil and stir.
2. In another bowl, mix egg with milk, salt and pepper and stir.
3. Sprinkle onion wedges with paprika and garlic powder, dip them in egg mix, then in bread crumbs mix, place in

your air fryer's basket, cook at 360 degrees F for 10 minutes, flip and cook for 5 minutes more.

4. Divide among plates and serve as a side dish.

Enjoy!

Nutrition: calories 200, fat 2, fiber 2, carbs 14, protein 7

Wild Rice Pilaf

Preparation time: 10 minutes **Cooking time:** 25 minutes
Servings: 12

Ingredients:

- 1 shallot, chopped
- 1 teaspoon garlic, minced
- A drizzle of olive oil
- 1 cup farro
- ¾ cup wild rice
- 4 cups chicken stock
- Salt and black pepper to the taste
- 1 tablespoon parsley, chopped
- ½ cup hazelnuts, toasted and chopped
- ¾ cup cherries, dried
- Chopped chives for serving

Directions:

1. In a dish that fits your air fryer, mix shallot with garlic, oil, faro, wild rice, stock, salt, pepper, parsley, hazelnuts and cherries, stir, place in your air fryer's basket and cook at 350 degrees F for 25 minutes.
2. Divide among plates and serve as a side dish.

Enjoy!

Nutrition: calories 142, fat 4, fiber 4, carbs 16, protein 4

Pumpkin Rice

Preparation time: 5 minutes **Cooking time:** 30 minutes
Servings: 4

Ingredients:

- 2 tablespoons olive oil
- 1 small yellow onion, chopped
- 2 garlic cloves, minced
- 12 ounces white rice
- 4 cups chicken stock
- 6 ounces pumpkin puree
- ½ teaspoon nutmeg
- 1 teaspoon thyme, chopped
- ½ teaspoon ginger, grated
- ½ teaspoon cinnamon powder
- ½ teaspoon allspice
- 4 ounces heavy cream

Directions:

1. In a dish that fits your air fryer, mix oil with onion, garlic, rice, stock, pumpkin puree, nutmeg, thyme, ginger, cinnamon, allspice and cream, stir well, place in

your air fryer's basket and cook at 360 degrees F for 30 minutes.

2. Divide among plates and serve as a side dish.

Enjoy!

Nutrition: calories 261, fat 6, fiber 7, carbs 29, protein 4

Colored Veggie Rice

Preparation time: 10 minutes **Cooking time:** 25 minutes
Servings: 4

Ingredients:

- 2 cups basmati rice
- 1 cup mixed carrots, peas, corn and green beans
- 2 cups water
- ½ teaspoon green chili, minced
- ½ teaspoon ginger, grated
- 3 garlic cloves, minced
- 2 tablespoons butter
- 1 teaspoon cinnamon powder
- 1 tablespoon cumin seeds
- 2 bay leaves
- 3 whole cloves
- 5 black peppercorns
- 2 whole cardamoms
- 1 tablespoon sugar
- Salt to the taste

Directions:

1. Put the water in a heat proof dish that fits your air fryer, add rice, mixed veggies, green chili, grated ginger, garlic cloves, cinnamon, cloves, butter, cumin seeds, bay leaves, cardamoms, black peppercorns, salt and sugar, stir, put in your air fryer's basket and cook at 370 degrees F for 25 minutes.
2. Divide among plates and serve as a side dish.

Enjoy!

Nutrition: calories 283, fat 4, fiber 8, carbs 34, protein 14

Potato Casserole

Preparation time: 15 minutes **Cooking time:** 40 minutes
Servings: 4

Ingredients:

- 3 pounds sweet potatoes, scrubbed
- ¼ cup milk
- ½ teaspoon nutmeg, ground
- 2 tablespoons white flour
- ¼ teaspoon allspice, ground
- Salt to the taste

For the topping:

- ½ cup almond flour
- ½ cup walnuts, soaked, drained and ground
- ¼ cup pecans, soaked, drained and ground
- ¼ cup coconut, shredded
- 1 tablespoon chia seeds
- ¼ cup sugar
- 1 teaspoon cinnamon powder
- 5 tablespoons butter

Directions:

1. Place potatoes in your air fryer's basket, prick them with a fork and cook at 360 degrees F for 30 minutes.
2. Meanwhile, in a bowl, mix almond flour with pecans, walnuts, ¼ cup coconut, ¼ cup sugar, chia seeds, 1 teaspoon cinnamon and the butter and stir everything.
3. Transfer potatoes to a cutting board, cool them, peel and place them in a baking dish that fits your air fryer.
4. Add milk, flour, salt, nutmeg and allspice and stir
5. Add crumble mix you've made earlier on top, place dish in your air fryer's basket and cook at 400 degrees F for 8 minutes.
6. Divide among plates and serve as a side dish.

Enjoy!

Nutrition: calories 162, fat 4, fiber 8, carbs 18, protein 4

Lemony Artichokes

Preparation time: 10 minutes **Cooking time:** 15 minutes
Servings: 4

Ingredients:

- 2 medium artichokes, trimmed and halved
- Cooking spray
- 2 tablespoons lemon juice
- Salt and black pepper to the taste

Directions:

1. Grease your air fryer with cooking spray, add artichokes, drizzle lemon juice and sprinkle salt and black pepper and cook them at 380 degrees F for 15 minutes.
2. Divide them on plates and serve as a side dish.

Enjoy!

Nutrition: calories 121, fat 3, fiber 6, carbs 9, protein 4

Cauliflower and Broccoli Delight

Preparation time: 10 minutes **Cooking time:** 7 minutes

Servings: 4

Ingredients:

- 2 cauliflower heads, florets separated and steamed
- 1 broccoli head, florets separated and steamed
- Zest from 1 orange, grated
- Juice from 1 orange
- A pinch of hot pepper flakes
- 4 anchovies
- 1 tablespoon capers, chopped
- Salt and black pepper to the taste
- 4 tablespoons olive oil

Directions:

1. In a bowl, mix orange zest with orange juice, pepper flakes, anchovies, capers salt, pepper and olive oil and whisk well.
2. Add broccoli and cauliflower, toss well, transfer them to your air fryer's basket and cook at 400 degrees F for 7 minutes.
3. Divide among plates and serve as a side dish with some of the orange vinaigrette drizzled on top.

Enjoy!

Nutrition: calories 300, fat 4, fiber 7, carbs 28, protein 4

Garlic Beet Wedges

Preparation time: 10 minutes **Cooking time:** 15 minutes
Servings: 4

Ingredients:

- 4 beets, washed, peeled and cut into large wedges
- 1 tablespoon olive oil
- Salt and black to the taste
- 2 garlic cloves, minced
- 1 teaspoon lemon juice

Directions:

1. In a bowl, mix beets with oil, salt, pepper, garlic and lemon juice, toss well, transfer to your air fryer's basket and cook them at 400 degrees F for 15 minutes.
2. Divide beets wedges on plates and serve as a side dish.

Enjoy!

Nutrition: calories 182, fat 6, fiber 3, carbs 8, protein 2

Fried Red Cabbage

Preparation time: 10 minutes **Cooking time:** 15 minutes
Servings: 4

Ingredients:

- 4 garlic cloves, minced
- ½ cup yellow onion, chopped
- 1 tablespoon olive oil
- 6 cups red cabbage, chopped
- 1 cup veggie stock
- 1 tablespoon apple cider vinegar
- 1 cup applesauce
- Salt and black pepper to the taste

Directions:

1. In a heat proof dish that fits your air fryer, mix cabbage with onion, garlic, oil, stock, vinegar, applesauce, salt and pepper, toss really well, place dish in your air fryer's basket and cook at 380 degrees F for 15 minutes.
2. Divide among plates and serve as a side dish.

Enjoy!

Nutrition: calories 172, fat 7, fiber 7, carbs 14, protein 5

Artichokes and Tarragon Sauce

Preparation time: 10 minutes **Cooking time:** 18 minutes
Servings: 4

Ingredients:

- 4 artichokes, trimmed
- 2 tablespoons tarragon, chopped
- 2 tablespoons chicken stock
- Lemon zest from 2 lemons, grated
- 2 tablespoons lemon juice
- 1 celery stalk, chopped
- ½ cup olive oil
- Salt to the taste

Directions:

1. In your food processor, mix tarragon, chicken stock, lemon zest, lemon juice, celery, salt and olive oil and pulse very well.
2. In a bowl, mix artichokes with tarragon and lemon sauce, toss well, transfer them to your air fryer's basket and cook at 380 degrees F for 18 minutes.
3. Divide artichokes on plates, drizzle the rest of the sauce all over and serve as a side dish.

Enjoy!

Nutrition: calories 215, fat 3, fiber 8, carbs 28, protein 6

Brussels Sprouts and Pomegranate Seeds Side Dish

Preparation time: 5 minutes **Cooking time:** 10 minutes

Servings: 4

Ingredients:

- 1 pound Brussels sprouts, trimmed and halved
- Salt and black pepper to the taste
- 1 cup pomegranate seeds
- ¼ cup pine nuts, toasted
- 1 tablespoons olive oil
- 2 tablespoons veggie stock

Directions:

1. In a heat proof dish that fits your air fryer, mix Brussels sprouts with salt, pepper, pomegranate seeds, pine nuts, oil and stock, stir, place in your air fryer's basket and cook at 390 degrees F for 10 minutes.
2. Divide among plates and serve as a side dish.

Enjoy!

Nutrition: calories 152, fat 4, fiber 7, carbs 12, protein 3

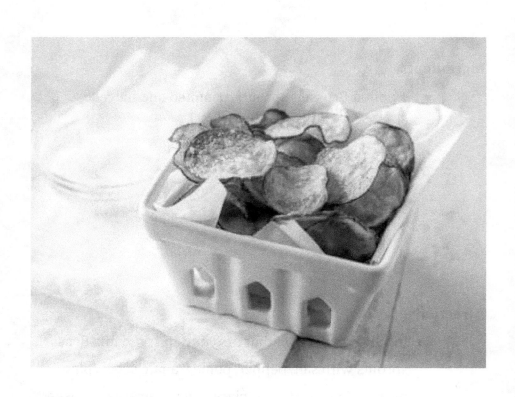

Crispy Brussels Sprouts and Potatoes

Preparation time: 10 minutes **Cooking time:** 8 minutes
Servings: 4

Ingredients:

- 1 and ½ pounds Brussels sprouts, washed and trimmed
- 1 cup new potatoes, chopped
- 1 and ½ tablespoons bread crumbs
- Salt and black pepper to the taste
- 1 and ½ tablespoons butter

Directions:

1. Put Brussels sprouts and potatoes in your air fryer's pan, add bread crumbs, salt, pepper and butter, toss well and cook at 400 degrees F for 8 minutes.
2. Divide among plates and serve as a side dish.

Enjoy!

Nutrition: calories 152, fat 3, fiber 7, carbs 17, protein 4

Coconut Chicken Bites

Preparation time: 10 minutes **Cooking time:** 13 minutes
Servings: 4

Ingredients:

- 2 teaspoons garlic powder
- 2 eggs
- Salt and black pepper to the taste
- ¾ cup panko bread crumbs
- ¾ cup coconut, shredded
- Cooking spray
- 8 chicken tenders

Directions:

1. In a bowl, mix eggs with salt, pepper and garlic powder and whisk well.
2. In another bowl, mix coconut with panko and stir well.
3. Dip chicken tenders in eggs mix and then coat in coconut one well.

4. Spray chicken bites with cooking spray, place them in your air fryer's basket and cook them at 350 degrees F for 10 minutes.

5. Arrange them on a platter and serve as an appetizer.

Enjoy!

Nutrition: calories 252, fat 4, fiber 2, carbs 14, protein 24

Buffalo Cauliflower Snack

Preparation time: 10 minutes **Cooking time:** 15 minutes

Servings: 4

Ingredients:

- 4 cups cauliflower florets
- 1 cup panko bread crumbs
- ¼ cup butter, melted
- ¼ cup buffalo sauce
- Mayonnaise for serving

Directions:

1. In a bowl, mix buffalo sauce with butter and whisk well.
2. Dip cauliflower florets in this mix and coat them in panko bread crumbs.
3. Place them in your air fryer's basket and cook at 350 degrees F for 15 minutes.
4. Arrange them on a platter and serve with mayo on the side.

Enjoy!

Nutrition: calories 241, fat 4, fiber 7, carbs 8, protein 4

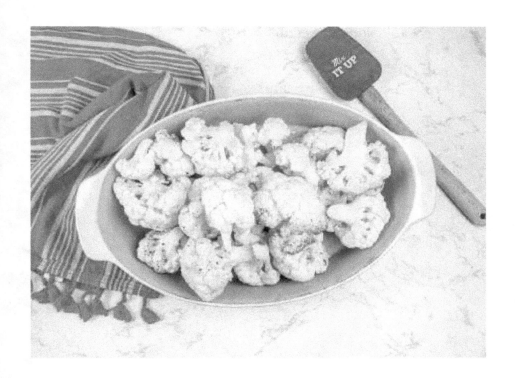

Banana Snack

Preparation time: 10 minutes **Cooking time:** 5 minutes
Servings: 8

Ingredients:

- 16 baking cups crust
- ¼ cup peanut butter
- ¾ cup chocolate chips
- 1 banana, peeled and sliced into 16 pieces
- 1 tablespoon vegetable oil

Directions:

1. Put chocolate chips in a small pot, heat up over low heat, stir until it melts and take off heat.
2. In a bowl, mix peanut butter with coconut oil and whisk well.
3. Spoon 1 teaspoon chocolate mix in a cup, add 1 banana slice and top with 1 teaspoon butter mix
4. Repeat with the rest of the cups, place them all into a dish that fits your air fryer, cook at 320 degrees F for 5 minutes, transfer to a freezer and keep there until you serve them as a snack.

Enjoy!

Nutrition: calories 70, fat 4, fiber 1, carbs 10, protein 1

Potato Spread

Preparation time: 10 minutes **Cooking time:** 10 minutes
Servings: 10

Ingredients:

- 19 ounces canned garbanzo beans, drained
- 1 cup sweet potatoes, peeled and chopped
- ¼ cup tahini
- 2 tablespoons lemon juice
- 1 tablespoon olive oil
- 5 garlic cloves, minced
- ½ teaspoon cumin, ground
- 2 tablespoons water
- A pinch of salt and white pepper

Directions:

1. Put potatoes in your air fryer's basket, cook them at 360 degrees F for 15 minutes, cool them down, peel, put them in your food processor and pulse well. basket,

2. Add sesame paste, garlic, beans, lemon juice, cumin, water and oil and pulse really well.

3. Add salt and pepper, pulse again, divide into bowls and serve.

Enjoy!

Nutrition: calories 200, fat 3, fiber 10, carbs 20, protein 11

Mexican Apple Snack

Preparation time: 10 minutes **Cooking time:** 5 minutes
Servings: 4

Ingredients:

- 3 big apples, cored, peeled and cubed
- 2 teaspoons lemon juice
- ¼ cup pecans, chopped
- ½ cup dark chocolate chips
- ½ cup clean caramel sauce

Directions:

1. In a bowl, mix apples with lemon juice, stir and transfer to a pan that fits your air fryer.
2. Add chocolate chips, pecans, drizzle the caramel sauce, toss, introduce in your air fryer and cook at 320 degrees F for 5 minutes.
3. Toss gently, divide into small bowls and serve right away as a snack.

Enjoy!

Nutrition: calories 200, fat 4, fiber 3, carbs 20, protein 3

Shrimp Muffins

Preparation time: 10 minutes **Cooking time:** 26 minutes

Servings: 6

Ingredients:

- 1 spaghetti squash, peeled and halved
- 2 tablespoons mayonnaise
- 1 cup mozzarella, shredded
- 8 ounces shrimp, peeled, cooked and chopped
- 1 and ½ cups panko
- 1 teaspoon parsley flakes
- 1 garlic clove, minced
- Salt and black pepper to the taste
- Cooking spray

Directions:

1. Put squash halves in your air fryer, cook at 350 degrees F for 16 minutes, leave aside to cool down and scrape flesh into a bowl.
2. Add salt, pepper, parsley flakes, panko, shrimp, mayo and mozzarella and stir well.

3. Spray a muffin tray that fits your air fryer with cooking spray and divide squash and shrimp mix in each cup.
4. Introduce in the fryer and cook at 360 degrees F for 10 minutes.
5. Arrange muffins on a platter and serve as a snack.

Enjoy!

Nutrition: calories 60, fat 2, fiber 0.4, carbs 4, protein 4

Zucchini Cakes

Preparation time: 10 minutes **Cooking time:** 12 minutes
Servings: 12

Ingredients:

- Cooking spray
- ½ cup dill, chopped
- 1 egg
- ½ cup whole wheat flour
- Salt and black pepper to the taste
- 1 yellow onion, chopped
- 2 garlic cloves, minced
- 3 zucchinis, grated

Directions:

1. In a bowl, mix zucchinis with garlic, onion, flour, salt, pepper, egg and dill, stir well, shape small patties out of this mix, spray them with cooking spray, place them in your air fryer's basket and cook at 370 degrees F for 6 minutes on each side.

2. Serve them as a snack right away.

Enjoy!

Nutrition: calories 60, fat 1, fiber 2, carbs 6, protein 2

Cauliflower Bars

Preparation time: 10 minutes **Cooking time:** 25 minutes

Servings: 12

Ingredients:

- 1 big cauliflower head, florets separated
- ½ cup mozzarella, shredded
- ¼ cup egg whites
- 1 teaspoon Italian seasoning
- Salt and black pepper to the taste

Directions:

1. Put cauliflower florets in your food processor, pulse well, spread on a lined baking sheet that fits your air fryer, introduce in the fryer and cook at 360 degrees F for 10 minutes.

2. Transfer cauliflower to a bowl, add salt, pepper, cheese, egg whites and Italian seasoning, stir really well, spread this into a rectangle pan that fits your air fryer, press well, introduce in the fryer and cook at 360 degrees F for 15 minutes more.

3. Cut into 12 bars, arrange them on a platter and serve as a snack

Enjoy!

Nutrition: calories 50, fat 1, fiber 2, carbs 3, protein 3

Pesto Crackers

Preparation time: 10 minutes **Cooking time:** 17 minutes
Servings: 6

Ingredients:
- ½ teaspoon baking powder
- Salt and black pepper to the taste
- 1 and ¼ cups flour
- ¼ teaspoon basil, dried
- 1 garlic clove, minced
- 2 tablespoons basil pesto
- 3 tablespoons butter

Directions:

1. In a bowl, mix salt, pepper, baking powder, flour, garlic, cayenne, basil, pesto and butter and stir until you obtain a dough.
2. Spread this dough on a lined baking sheet that fits your air fryer, introduce in the fryer at 325 degrees F and bake for 17 minutes.
3. Leave aside to cool down, cut crackers and serve them as a snack.

Enjoy!

Nutrition: calories 200, fat 20, fiber 1, carbs 4, protein 7

Pumpkin Muffins

Preparation time: 10 minutes **Cooking time:** 15 minutes
Servings: 18

Ingredients:

- ¼ cup butter
- ¾ cup pumpkin puree
- 2 tablespoons flaxseed meal
- ¼ cup flour
- ½ cup sugar
- ½ teaspoon nutmeg, ground
- 1 teaspoon cinnamon powder
- ½ teaspoon baking soda
- 1 egg
- ½ teaspoon baking powder

Directions:

1. In a bowl, mix butter with pumpkin puree and egg and blend well.
2. Add flaxseed meal, flour, sugar, baking soda, baking powder, nutmeg and cinnamon and stir well.

3. Spoon this into a muffin pan that fits your fryer introduce in the fryer at 350 degrees F and bake for 15 minutes.

4. Serve muffins cold as a snack.

Enjoy!

Nutrition: calories 50, fat 3, fiber 1, carbs 2, protein 2

Zucchini Chips

Preparation time: 10 minutes **Cooking time:** 1 hour **Servings:** 6

Ingredients:

- 3 zucchinis, thinly sliced
- Salt and black pepper to the taste
- 2 tablespoons olive oil
- 2 tablespoons balsamic vinegar

Directions:

1. In a bowl, mix oil with vinegar, salt and pepper and whisk well.
2. Add zucchini slices, toss to coat well, introduce in your air fryer and cook at 200 degrees F for 1 hour.
3. Serve zucchini chips cold as a snack.

Enjoy!

Nutrition: calories 40, fat 3, fiber 7, carbs 3, protein 7

Beef Jerky Snack

Preparation time: 2 hours **Cooking time:** 1 hour and 30 minutes
Servings: 6

Ingredients:

- 2 cups soy sauce
- ½ cup Worcestershire sauce
- 2 tablespoons black peppercorns
- 2 tablespoons black pepper
- 2 pounds beef round, sliced

Directions:

1. In a bowl, mix soy sauce with black peppercorns, black pepper and Worcestershire sauce and whisk well.
2. Add beef slices, toss to coat and leave aside in the fridge for 6 hours.
3. Introduce beef rounds in your air fryer and cook them at 370 degrees F for 1 hour and 30 minutes.
4. Transfer to a bowl and serve cold.

Enjoy!

Nutrition: calories 300, fat 12, fiber 4, carbs 3, protein 8

Honey Party Wings

Preparation time: 1 hour and 10 minutes **Cooking time:** 12 minutes **Servings:** 8

Ingredients:

- 16 chicken wings, halved
- 2 tablespoons soy sauce
- 2 tablespoons honey
- Salt and black pepper to the taste
- 2 tablespoons lime juice

Directions:

1. In a bowl, mix chicken wings with soy sauce, honey, salt, pepper and lime juice, toss well and keep in the fridge for 1 hour.
2. Transfer chicken wings to your air fryer and cook them at 360 degrees F for 12 minutes, flipping them halfway.
3. Arrange them on a platter and serve as an appetizer.

Enjoy!

Nutrition: calories 211, fat 4, fiber 7, carbs 14, protein 3

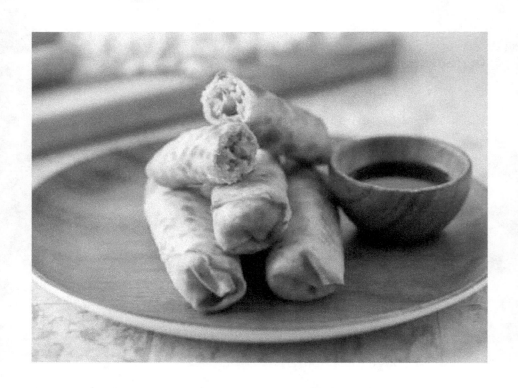

Salmon Party Patties

Preparation time: 10 minutes **Cooking time:** 22 minutes

Servings: 4

Ingredients:

- 3 big potatoes, boiled, drained and mashed
- 1 big salmon fillet, skinless, boneless
- 2 tablespoons parsley, chopped
- 2 tablespoon dill, chopped
- Salt and black pepper to the taste
- 1 egg
- 2 tablespoons bread crumbs
- Cooking spray

Directions:

1. Place salmon in your air fryer's basket and cook for 10 minutes at 360 degrees F.
2. Transfer salmon to a cutting board, cool it down, flake it and put it in a bowl.
3. Add mashed potatoes, salt, pepper, dill, parsley, egg and bread crumbs, stir well and shape 8 patties out of this mix.
4. Place salmon patties in your air fryer's basket, spry them with cooking oil, cook at 360 degrees F for 12 minutes, flipping them halfway, transfer them to a platter and serve as an appetizer.

Enjoy!

Nutrition: calories 231, fat 3, fiber 7, carbs 14, protein 4

Banana Chips

Preparation time: 10 minutes **Cooking time:** 15 minutes

Servings: 4

Ingredients:

- 4 bananas, peeled and sliced
- A pinch of salt
- ½ teaspoon turmeric powder
- ½ teaspoon chaat masala
- 1 teaspoon olive oil

Directions:

1. In a bowl, mix banana slices with salt, turmeric, chaat masala and oil, toss and leave aside for 10 minutes.
2. Transfer banana slices to your preheated air fryer at 360 degrees F and cook them for 15 minutes flipping them once.
3. Serve as a snack.

Enjoy!

Nutrition: calories 121, fat 1, fiber 2, carbs 3, protein 3

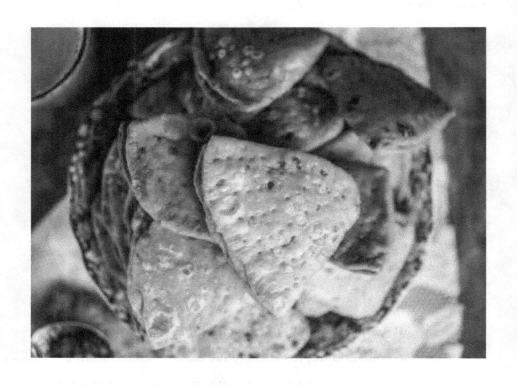

Spring Rolls

Preparation time: 10 minutes **Cooking time:** 25 minutes
Servings: 8

Ingredients:

- 2 cups green cabbage, shredded
- 2 yellow onions, chopped
- 1 carrot, grated
- ½ chili pepper, minced
- 1 tablespoon ginger, grated
- 3 garlic cloves, minced
- 1 teaspoon sugar
- Salt and black pepper to the taste
- 1 teaspoon soy sauce
- 2 tablespoons olive oil
- 10 spring roll sheets
- 2 tablespoons corn flour
- 2 tablespoons water

Directions:

1. Heat up a pan with the oil over medium heat, add
   cabbage, onions, carrots, chili pepper, ginger, garlic,

sugar, salt, pepper and soy sauce, stir well, cook for 2-3 minutes, take off heat and cool down.

2. Cut spring roll sheets in squares, divide cabbage mix on each and roll them.
3. In a bowl, mix corn flour with water, stir well and seal spring rolls with this mix.
4. Place spring rolls in your air fryer's basket and cook them at 360 degrees F for 10 minutes.
5. Flip roll and cook them for 10 minutes more.
6. Arrange on a platter and serve them as an appetizer.

Enjoy!

Nutrition: calories 214, fat 4, fiber 4, carbs 12, protein 4

Crispy Radish Chips

Preparation time: 10 minutes **Cooking time:** 10 minutes
Servings: 4

Ingredients:
- Cooking spray
- 15 radishes, sliced
- Salt and black pepper to the taste
- 1 tablespoon chives, chopped

Directions:
1. Arrange radish slices in your air fryer's basket, spray them with cooking oil, season with salt and black pepper to the taste, cook them at 350 degrees F for 10 minutes, flipping them halfway, transfer to bowls and serve with chives sprinkled on top.

Enjoy!

Nutrition: calories 80, fat 1, fiber 1, carbs 1, protein 1

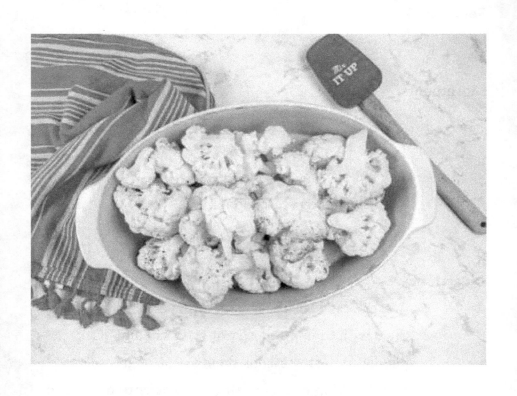

Crab Sticks

Preparation time: 10 minutes **Cooking time:** 12 minutes

Servings: 4

Ingredients:
- 10 crabsticks, halved
- 2 teaspoons sesame oil
- 2 teaspoons Cajun seasoning

Directions:
1. Put crab sticks in a bowl, add sesame oil and Cajun seasoning, toss, transfer them to your air fryer's basket and cook at 350 degrees F for 12 minutes.
   Arrange on a platter and serve as an appetizer.

Enjoy!

Nutrition: calories 110, fat 0, fiber 1, carbs 4, protein 2

Air Fried Dill Pickles

Preparation time: 10 minutes **Cooking time:** 5 minutes

Servings: 4

Ingredients:

- 16 ounces jarred dill pickles, cut into wedges and pat dried
- ½ cup white flour
- 1 egg
- ¼ cup milk
- ½ teaspoon garlic powder
- ½ teaspoon sweet paprika
- Cooking spray
- ¼ cup ranch sauce

Directions:

1. In a bowl, combine milk with egg and whisk well.
2. In a second bowl, mix flour with salt, garlic powder and paprika and stir as well
3. Dip pickles in flour, then in egg mix and again in flour and place them in your air fryer.

4. Grease them with cooking spray, cook pickle wedges at 400 degrees F for 5 minutes, transfer to a bowl and serve with ranch sauce on the side.

Enjoy!

Nutrition: calories 109, fat 2, fiber 2, carbs 10, protein 4

Chickpeas Snack

Preparation time: 10 minutes **Cooking time:** 10 minutes
Servings: 4

Ingredients:

- 15 ounces canned chickpeas, drained
- ½ teaspoon cumin, ground
- 1 tablespoon olive oil
- 1 teaspoon smoked paprika
- Salt and black pepper to the taste

Directions:

1. In a bowl, mix chickpeas with oil, cumin, paprika, salt and pepper, toss to coat, place them in your fryer's basket and cook at 390 degrees F for 10 minutes.
2. Divide into bowls and serve as a snack.

Enjoy!

Nutrition: calories 140, fat 1, fiber 6, carbs 20, protein 6

Sausage Balls

Preparation time: 10 minutes **Cooking time:** 15 minutes
Servings: 9

Ingredients:

- 4 ounces sausage meat, ground
- Salt and black pepper to the taste
- 1 teaspoon sage
- ½ teaspoon garlic, minced
- 1 small onion, chopped
- 3 tablespoons breadcrumbs

Directions:

1. In a bowl, mix sausage with salt, pepper, sage, garlic, onion and breadcrumbs, stir well and shape small balls out of this mix.
2. Put them in your air fryer's basket, cook at 360 degrees F for 15 minutes, divide into bowls and serve as a snack.

Enjoy!

Nutrition: calories 130, fat 7, fiber 1, carbs 13, protein 4

Chicken Dip

Preparation time: 10 minutes **Cooking time:** 25 minutes
Servings: 10

Ingredients:

- 3 tablespoons butter, melted
- 1 cup yogurt
- 12 ounces cream cheese
- 2 cups chicken meat, cooked and shredded
- 2 teaspoons curry powder
- 4 scallions, chopped
- 6 ounces Monterey jack cheese, grated
- 1/3 cup raisins
- ¼ cup cilantro, chopped
- ½ cup almonds, sliced
- Salt and black pepper to the taste
- ½ cup chutney

Directions:

1. In a bowl mix cream cheese with yogurt and whisk using your mixer.

117

2. Add curry powder, scallions, chicken meat, raisins, cheese, cilantro, salt and pepper and stir everything.
3. Spread this into a baking dish that fist your air fryer, sprinkle almonds on top, place in your air fryer, bake at 300 degrees for 25 minutes, divide into bowls, top with chutney and serve as an appetizer.

Enjoy!

Nutrition: calories 240, fat 10, fiber 2, carbs 24, protein 12

Sweet Popcorn

Preparation time: 5 minutes **Cooking time:** 10 minutes

Servings: 4

Ingredients:

- 2 tablespoons corn kernels
- 2 and ½ tablespoons butter
- 2 ounces brown sugar

Directions:

1. Put corn kernels in your air fryer's pan, cook at 400 degrees F for 6 minutes, transfer them to a tray, spread and leave aside for now.
2. Heat up a pan over low heat, add butter, melt it, add sugar and stir until it dissolves.
3. Add popcorn, toss to coat, take off heat and spread on the tray again.
4. Cool down, divide into bowls and serve as a snack.

Enjoy!

Nutrition: calories 70, fat 0.2, fiber 0, carbs 1, protein 1

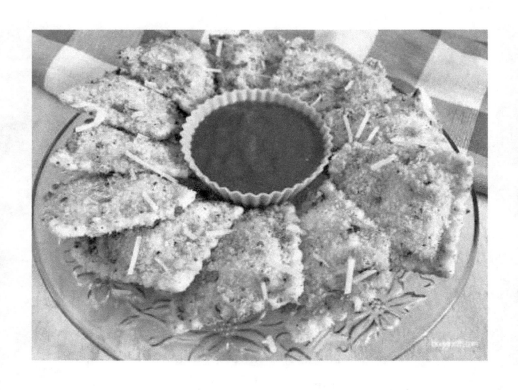

120

Apple Chips

Preparation time: 10 minutes **Cooking time:** 10 minutes
Servings: 2

Ingredients:

- 1 apple, cored and sliced
- A pinch of salt
- ½ teaspoon cinnamon powder
- 1 tablespoon white sugar

Directions:

1. In a bowl, mix apple slices with salt, sugar and cinnamon, toss, transfer to your air fryer's basket, cook for 10 minutes at 390 degrees F flipping once.
2. Divide apple chips in bowls and serve as a snack.

Enjoy!

Nutrition: calories 70, fat 0, fiber 4, carbs 3, protein 1

Bread Sticks

Preparation time: 10 minutes **Cooking time:** 10 minutes

Servings: 2

Ingredients:

- 4 bread slices, each cut into 4 sticks
- 2 eggs
- ¼ cup milk
- 1 teaspoon cinnamon powder
- 1 tablespoon honey
- ¼ cup brown sugar
- A pinch of nutmeg

Directions:

1. In a bowl, mix eggs with milk, brown sugar, cinnamon, nutmeg and honey and whisk well.
2. Dip bread sticks in this mix, place them in your air fryer's basket and cook at 360 degrees F for 10 minutes.
3. Divide bread sticks into bowls and serve as a snack.

Enjoy!

Nutrition: calories 140, fat 1, fiber 4, carbs 8, protein 4

Crispy Shrimp

Preparation time: 10 minutes **Cooking time:** 5 minutes

Servings: 4

Ingredients:

- 12 big shrimp, deveined and peeled
- 2 egg whites
- 1 cup coconut, shredded
- 1 cup panko bread crumbs
- 1 cup white flour
- Salt and black pepper to the taste

Directions:

1. In a bowl, mix panko with coconut and stir.
2. Put flour, salt and pepper in a second bowl and whisk egg whites in a third one.
3. Dip shrimp in flour, egg whites mix and coconut, place them all in your air fryer's basket, cook at 350 degrees F for 10 minutes flipping halfway.
4. Arrange on a platter and serve as an appetizer.

Enjoy!

Nutrition: calories 140, fat 4, fiber 0, carbs 3, protein 4

Cajun Shrimp Appetizer

Preparation time: 10 minutes **Cooking time:** 5 minutes
Servings: 2

Ingredients:

- 20 tiger shrimp, peeled and deveined
- Salt and black pepper to the taste
- ½ teaspoon old bay seasoning
- 1 tablespoon olive oil
- ¼ teaspoon smoked paprika

Directions:

1. In a bowl, mix shrimp with oil, salt, pepper, old bay seasoning and paprika and toss to coat.
2. Place shrimp in your air fryer's basket and cook at 390 degrees F for 5 minutes.
3. Arrange them on a platter and serve as an appetizer.

Enjoy!

Nutrition: calories 162, fat 6, fiber 4, carbs 8, protein 14

Crispy Fish Sticks

Preparation time: 10 minutes **Cooking time:** 12 minutes
Servings: 2

Ingredients:

- 4 ounces bread crumbs
- 4 tablespoons olive oil
- 1 egg, whisked
- 4 white fish filets, boneless, skinless and cut into medium sticks
- Salt and black pepper to the taste

Directions:

1. In a bowl, mix bread crumbs with oil and stir well.
2. Put egg in a second bowl, add salt and pepper and whisk well.
3. Dip fish stick in egg and them in bread crumb mix, place them in your air fryer's basket and cook at 360 degrees F for 12 minutes.
4. Arrange fish sticks on a platter and serve as an appetizer.

Enjoy!

Nutrition: calories 160, fat 3, fiber 5, carbs 12, protein 3

Fish Nuggets

Preparation time: 10 minutes **Cooking time:** 12 minutes
Servings: 4

Ingredients:

- 28 ounces fish fillets, skinless and cut into medium pieces
- Salt and black pepper to the taste
- 5 tablespoons flour
- 1 egg, whisked
- 5 tablespoons water
- 3 ounces panko bread crumbs
- 1 tablespoon garlic powder
- 1 tablespoon smoked paprika
- 4 tablespoons homemade mayonnaise
- Lemon juice from ½ lemon
- 1 teaspoon dill, dried
- Cooking spray

Directions:

1. In a bowl, mix flour with water and stir well.
2. Add egg, salt and pepper and whisk well.

3. In a second bowl, mix panko with garlic powder and paprika and stir well.
4. Dip fish pieces in flour and egg mix and then in panko mix, place them in your air fryer's basket, spray them with cooking oil and cook at 400 degrees F for 12 minutes.
5. Meanwhile, in a bowl mix mayo with dill and lemon juice and whisk well.
6. Arrange fish nuggets on a platter and serve with dill mayo on the side.

Enjoy!

Nutrition: calories 332, fat 12, fiber 6, carbs 17, protein 15

Shrimp and Chestnut Rolls

Preparation time: 10 minutes **Cooking time:** 15 minutes

Servings: 4

Ingredients:

- ½ pound already cooked shrimp, chopped
- 8 ounces water chestnuts, chopped
- ½ pounds shiitake mushrooms, chopped
- 2 cups cabbage, chopped
- 2 tablespoons olive oil
- 1 garlic clove, minced
- 1 teaspoon ginger, grated
- 3 scallions, chopped
- Salt and black pepper to the taste
- 1 tablespoon water
- 1 egg yolk
- 6 spring roll wrappers

Directions:

1. Heat up a pan with the oil over medium high heat, add cabbage, shrimp, chestnuts, mushrooms, garlic, ginger, scallions, salt and pepper, stir and cook for 2 minutes.

2. In a bowl, mix egg with water and stir well.

3. Arrange roll wrappers on a working surface, divide shrimp and veggie mix on them, seal edges with egg wash, place them all in your air fryer's basket, cook at 360 degrees F for 15 minutes, transfer to a platter and serve as an appetizer.

Enjoy!

Nutrition: calories 140, fat 3, fiber 1, carbs 12, protein 3

Seafood Appetizer

Preparation time: 10 minutes **Cooking time:** 25 minutes
Servings: 4

Ingredients:

- ½ cup yellow onion, chopped
- 1 cup green bell pepper, chopped
- 1 cup celery, chopped
- 1 cup baby shrimp, peeled and deveined
- 1 cup crabmeat, flaked
- 1 cup homemade mayonnaise
- 1 teaspoon Worcestershire sauce
- Salt and black pepper to the taste
- 2 tablespoons bread crumbs
- 1 tablespoon butter
- 1 teaspoon sweet paprika

Directions:

1. In a bowl, mix shrimp with crab meat, bell pepper, onion, mayo, celery, salt and pepper and stir.
2. Add Worcestershire sauce, stir again and pour everything into a baking dish that fits your air fryer.

3. Sprinkle bread crumbs and add butter, introduce in your air fryer and cook at 320 degrees F for 25 minutes, shaking halfway.

4. Divide into bowl and serve with paprika sprinkled on top as an appetizer.

Enjoy!

Nutrition: calories 200, fat 1, fiber 2, carbs 5, protein 1

Salmon Meatballs

Preparation time: 10 minutes **Cooking time:** 12 minutes
Servings: 4

Ingredients:
- 3 tablespoons cilantro, minced
- 1 pound salmon, skinless and chopped
- 1 small yellow onion, chopped
- 1 egg white
- Salt and black pepper to the taste
- 2 garlic cloves, minced
- ½ teaspoon paprika
- ¼ cup panko
- ½ teaspoon oregano, ground
- Cooking spray

Directions:
1. In your food processor, mix salmon with onion, cilantro, egg white, garlic cloves, salt, pepper, paprika and oregano and stir well.
2. Add panko, blend again and shape meatballs from this mix using your palms.

3. Place them in your air fryer's basket, spray them with cooking spray and cook at 320 degrees F for 12 minutes shaking the fryer halfway.
4. Arrange meatballs on a platter and serve them as an appetizer.

Enjoy!

Nutrition: calories 289, fat 12, fiber 3, carbs 22, protein 23

Easy Chicken Wings

Preparation time: 10 minutes **Cooking time:** 1 hours **Servings:** 2

Ingredients:

- 16 pieces chicken wings
- Salt and black pepper to the taste
- ¼ cup butter
- ¾ cup potato starch
- ¼ cup honey
- 4 tablespoons garlic, minced

Directions:

1. In a bowl, mix chicken wings with salt, pepper and potato starch, toss well, transfer to your air fryer's basket, cook them at 380 degrees F for 25 minutes and at 400 degrees F for 5 minutes more.
2. Meanwhile, heat up a pan with the butter over medium high heat, melt it, add garlic, stir, cook for 5 minutes and then mix with salt, pepper and honey.
3. Whisk well, cook over medium heat for 20 minutes and take off heat.
4. Arrange chicken wings on a platter, drizzle honey sauce all over and serve as an appetizer.

Enjoy!

Nutrition: calories 244, fat 7, fiber 3, carbs 19, protein 8

Chicken Breast Rolls

Preparation time: 10 minutes **Cooking time:** 22 minutes
Servings: 4

Ingredients:

- 2 cups baby spinach
- 4 chicken breasts, boneless and skinless
- 1 cup sun dried tomatoes, chopped
- Salt and black pepper to the taste
- 1 and ½ tablespoons Italian seasoning
- 4 mozzarella slices
- A drizzle of olive oil

Directions:

1. Flatten chicken breasts using a meat tenderizer, divide tomatoes, mozzarella and spinach, season with salt, pepper and Italian seasoning, roll and seal them.
2. Place them in your air fryer's basket, drizzle some oil over them and cook at 375 degrees F for 17 minutes, flipping once.
3. Arrange chicken rolls on a platter and serve them as an appetizer.

Enjoy!

Nutrition: calories 300, fat 1, fiber 4, carbs 7, protein 10

Crispy Chicken Breast Sticks

Preparation time: 10 minutes **Cooking time:** 16 minutes
Servings: 4

Ingredients:

- ¾ cup white flour
- 1 pound chicken breast, skinless, boneless and cut into medium sticks
- 1 teaspoon sweet paprika
- 1 cup panko bread crumbs
- 1 egg, whisked
- Salt and black pepper to the taste
- ½ tablespoon olive oil
- Zest from 1 lemon, grated

Directions:

1. In a bowl, mix paprika with flour, salt, pepper and lemon zest and stir.
2. Put whisked egg in another bowl and the panko breadcrumbs in a third one.
3. Dredge chicken pieces in flour, egg and panko and place them in your lined air fryer's basket, drizzle the oil over them, cook at 400 degrees F for 8 minutes, flip and cook for 8 more minutes.
4. Arrange them on a platter and serve as a snack.

Enjoy!

Nutrition: calories 254, fat 4, fiber 7, carbs 20, protein 22

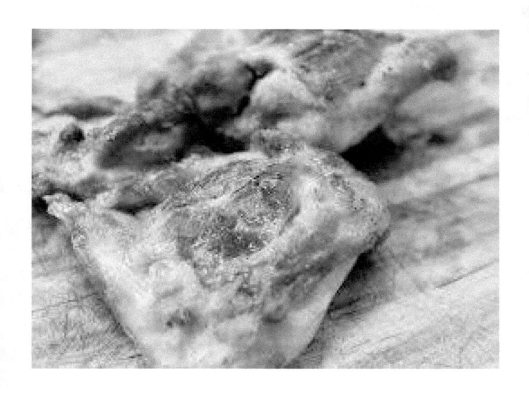

Beef Roll s

Preparation time: 10 minutes **Cooking time:** 14 minutes

Servings: 4

Ingredients:

- 2 pounds beef steak, opened and flattened with a meat tenderizer
- Salt and black pepper to the taste
- 1 cup baby spinach
- 3 ounces red bell pepper, roasted and chopped
- 6 slices provolone cheese
- 3 tablespoons pesto

Directions:

1. Arrange flattened beef steak on a cutting board, spread pesto all over, add cheese in a single layer, add bell peppers, spinach, salt and pepper to the taste.
2. Roll your steak, secure with toothpicks, season again with salt and pepper, place roll in your air fryer's basket and cook at 400 degrees F for 14 minutes, rotating roll halfway.
3. Leave aside to cool down, cut into 2 inch smaller rolls, arrange on a platter and serve them as an appetizer.

Enjoy!

Nutrition: calories 230, fat 1, fiber 3, carbs 12, protein 10

Empanadas

Preparation time: 10 minutes **Cooking time:** 25 minutes

Servings: 4

Ingredients:

- 1 package empanada shells
- 1 tablespoon olive oil
- 1 pound beef meat, ground
- 1 yellow onion, chopped
- Salt and black pepper to the taste
- 2 garlic cloves, minced
- ½ teaspoon cumin, ground
- ¼ cup tomato salsa
- 1 egg yolk whisked with 1 tablespoon water
- 1 green bell pepper, chopped

Directions:

1. Heat up a pan with the oil over medium high heat, add beef and brown on all sides.
2. Add onion, garlic, salt, pepper, bell pepper and tomato salsa, stir and cook for 15 minutes.

3. Divide cooked meat in empanada shells, brush them with egg wash and seal.
4. Place them in your air fryer's steamer basket and cook at 350 degrees F for 10 minutes.
5. Arrange on a platter and serve as an appetizer.

Enjoy!

Nutrition: calories 274, fat 17, fiber 14, carbs 20, protein 7

Greek Lamb Meatballs

Preparation time: 10 minutes **Cooking time:** 8 minutes
Servings: 10

Ingredients:

- 4 ounces lamb meat, minced
- Salt and black pepper to the taste
- 1 slice of bread, toasted and crumbled
- 2 tablespoons feta cheese, crumbled
- ½ tablespoon lemon peel, grated
- 1 tablespoon oregano, chopped

Directions:

1. In a bowl, combine meat with bread crumbs, salt, pepper, feta, oregano and lemon peel, stir well, shape 10 meatballs and place them in you air fryer.
2. Cook at 400 degrees F for 8 minutes, arrange them on a platter and serve as an appetizer.

Enjoy!

Nutrition: calories 234, fat 12, fiber 2, carbs 20, protein 30

Beef Party Rolls

Preparation time: 10 minutes **Cooking time:** 15 minutes

Servings: 4

Ingredients:

- 14 ounces beef stock
- 7 ounces white wine
- 4 beef cutlets
- Salt and black pepper to the taste
- 8 sage leaves
- 4 ham slices
- 1 tablespoon butter, melted

Directions:

1. Heat up a pan with the stock over medium high heat, add wine, cook until it reduces, take off heat and divide into small bowls
2. Season cutlets with salt and pepper, cover with sage and roll each in ham slices.
3. Brush rolls with butter, place them in your air fryer's basket and cook at 400 degrees F for 15 minutes.

4. Arrange rolls on a platter and serve them with the gravy on the side.

Enjoy!

Nutrition: calories 260, fat 12, fiber 1, carbs 22, protein 21

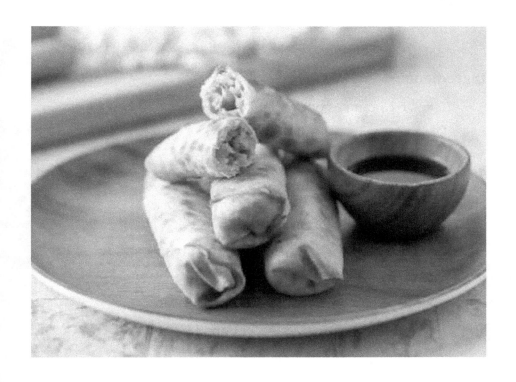

Pork Rolls

Preparation time: 10 minutes **Cooking time:** 40 minutes

Servings: 4

Ingredients:

- 1 15 ounces pork fillet
- ½ teaspoon chili powder
- 1 teaspoon cinnamon powder
- 1 garlic clove, minced
- Salt and black pepper to the taste
- 2 tablespoons olive oil
- 1 and ½ teaspoon cumin, ground
- 1 red onion, chopped
- 3 tablespoons parsley, chopped

Directions:

1. In a bowl, mix cinnamon with garlic, salt, pepper, chili powder, oil, onion, parsley and cumin and stir well
2. Put pork fillet on a cutting board, flatten it using a meat tenderizer. And use a meat tenderizer to flatten it.

3. Spread onion mix on pork, roll tight, cut into medium rolls, place them in your preheated air fryer at 360 degrees F and cook them for 35 minutes.

4. Arrange them on a platter and serve as an appetizer

Enjoy!

Nutrition: calories 304, fat 12, fiber 1, carbs 15, protein 23

Beef Patties

Preparation time: 10 minutes **Cooking time:** 8 minutes

Servings: 4

Ingredients:

- 14 ounces beef, minced
- 2 tablespoons ham, cut into strips
- 1 leek, chopped
- 3 tablespoons bread crumbs
- Salt and black pepper to the taste
- ½ teaspoon nutmeg, ground

Directions:

1. In a bowl, mix beef with leek, salt, pepper, ham, breadcrumbs and nutmeg, stir well and shape small patties out of this mix.
2. Place them in your air fryer's basket, cook at 400 degrees F for 8 minutes, arrange on a platter and serve as an appetizer.

Enjoy!

Nutrition: calories 260, fat 12, fiber 3, carbs 12, protein 21

Roasted Bell Pepper Rolls

Preparation time: 10 minutes **Cooking time:** 10 minutes **Servings:** 8

Ingredients:

- 1 yellow bell pepper, halved
- 1 orange bell pepper, halved
- Salt and black pepper to the taste
- 4 ounces feta cheese, crumbled
- 1 green onion, chopped
- 2 tablespoons oregano, chopped

Directions:

1. In a bowl, mix cheese with onion, oregano, salt and pepper and whisk well.
2. Place bell pepper halves in your air fryer's basket, cook at 400 degrees F for 10 minutes, transfer to a cutting board, cool down and peel.
3. Divide cheese mix on each bell pepper half, roll, secure with toothpicks, arrange on a platter and serve as an appetizer.

Enjoy!

Nutrition: calories 170, fat 1, fiber 2, carbs 8, protein 5

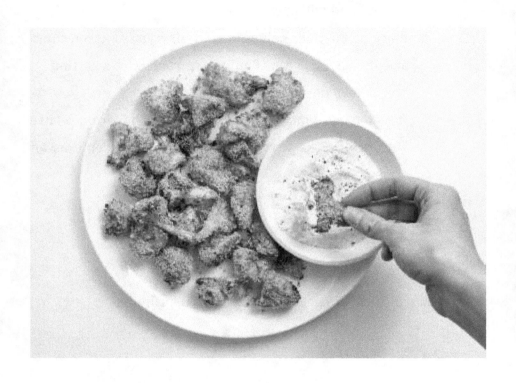

Stuffed Peppers

Preparation time: 10 minutes **Cooking time:** 8 minutes

Servings: 8

Ingredients:

- 8 small bell peppers, tops cut off and seeds removed
- 1 tablespoon olive oil
- Salt and black pepper to the taste
- 3.5 ounces goat cheese, cut into 8 pieces

Directions:

1. In a bowl, mix cheese with oil with salt and pepper and toss to coat.
2. Stuff each pepper with goat cheese, place them in your air fryer's basket, cook at 400 degrees F for 8 minutes, arrange on a platter and serve as an appetizer.

Enjoy!

Nutrition: calories 120, fat 1, fiber 1, carbs 12, protein 8

Herbed Tomatoes Appetizer

Preparation time: 10 minutes **Cooking time:** 20 minutes
Servings: 2

Ingredients:

- 2 tomatoes, halved
- Cooking spray
- Salt and black pepper to the taste
- 1 teaspoon parsley, dried
- 1 teaspoon basil, dried
- 1 teaspoon oregano, dried
- 1 teaspoon rosemary, dried

Directions:

1. Spray tomato halves with cooking oil, season with salt, pepper, parsley, basil, oregano and rosemary over them.
2. Place them in your air fryer's basket and cook at 320 degrees F for 20 minutes.
3. Arrange them on a platter and serve as an appetizer.

Enjoy!

Nutrition: calories 100, fat 1, fiber 1, carbs 4, protein 1

Olives Balls

Preparation time: 10 minutes **Cooking time:** 4 minutes
Servings: 6

Ingredients:

- 8 black olives, pitted and minced
- Salt and black pepper to the taste
- 2 tablespoons sun dried tomato pesto
- 14 pepperoni slices, chopped
- 4 ounces cream cheese
- 1 tablespoons basil, chopped

Directions:

1. In a bowl, mix cream cheese with salt, pepper, basil, pepperoni, pesto and black olives, stir well and shape small balls out of this mix.
2. Place them in your air fryer's basket, cook at 350 degrees F for 4 minutes, arrange on a platter and serve as a snack.

Enjoy!

Nutrition: calories 100, fat 1, fiber 0, carbs 8, protein 3

Jalapeno Balls

Preparation time: 10 minutes **Cooking time:** 4 minutes **Servings:** 3

Ingredients:

- 3 bacon slices, cooked and crumbled
- 3 ounces cream cheese
- ¼ teaspoon onion powder
- Salt and black pepper to the taste
- 1 jalapeno pepper, chopped
- ½ teaspoon parsley, dried
- ¼ teaspoon garlic powder

Directions:

1. In a bowl, mix cream cheese with jalapeno pepper, onion and garlic powder, parsley, bacon salt and pepper and stir well.
2. Shape small balls out of this mix, place them in your air fryer's basket, cook at 350 degrees F for 4 minutes, arrange on a platter and serve as an appetizer.

Enjoy!

Nutrition: calories 172, fat 4, fiber 1, carbs 12, protein 5

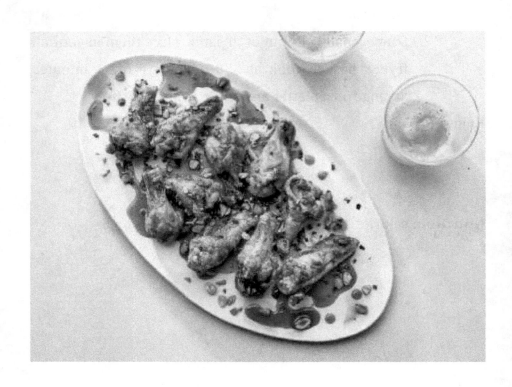

Wrapped Shrimp

Preparation time: 10 minutes **Cooking time:** 8 minutes **Servings:** 16

Ingredients:

- 2 tablespoons olive oil
- 10 ounces already cooked shrimp, peeled and deveined
- 1 tablespoons mint, chopped
- 1/3 cup blackberries, ground
- 11 prosciutto sliced
- 1/3 cup red wine

Directions:

1. Wrap each shrimp in a prosciutto slices, drizzle the oil over them, rub well, place in your preheated air fryer at 390 degrees F and fry them for 8 minutes.
2. Meanwhile, heat up a pan with ground blackberries over medium heat, add mint and wine, stir, cook for 3 minutes and take off heat.
3. Arrange shrimp on a platter, drizzle blackberries sauce over them and serve as an appetizer.

Enjoy!

Nutrition: calories 224, fat 12, fiber 2, carbs 12, protein 14

Broccoli Patties

Preparation time: 10 minutes **Cooking time:** 10 minutes
Servings: 12

Ingredients:

- 4 cups broccoli florets
- 1 and ½ cup almond flour
- 1 teaspoon paprika
- Salt and black pepper to the taste
- 2 eggs
- ¼ cup olive oil
- 2 cups cheddar cheese, grated
- 1 teaspoon garlic powder
- ½ teaspoon apple cider vinegar
- ½ teaspoon baking soda

Directions:

1. Put broccoli florets in your food processor, add salt and pepper, blend well and transfer to a bowl.
2. Add almond flour, salt, pepper, paprika, garlic powder, baking soda, cheese, oil, eggs and vinegar, stir well and shape 12 patties out of this mix.

3. Place them in your preheated air fryer's basket and cook at 350 degrees F for 10 minutes.

4. Arrange patties on a platter and serve as an appetizer.

Enjoy!

Nutrition: calories 203, fat 12, fiber 2, carbs 14, protein 2

Different Stuffed Peppers

Preparation time: 10 minutes **Cooking time:** 20 minutes
Servings: 6

Ingredients:

- 1 pound mini bell peppers, halved
- Salt and black pepper to the taste
- 1 teaspoon garlic powder
- 1 teaspoon sweet paprika
- ½ teaspoon oregano, dried
- ¼ teaspoon red pepper flakes
- 1 pound beef meat, ground
- 1 and ½ cups cheddar cheese, shredded
- 1 tablespoons chili powder
- 1 teaspoon cumin, ground
- Sour cream for serving

Directions:

1. In a bowl, mix chili powder with paprika, salt, pepper, cumin, oregano, pepper flakes and garlic powder and stir.

2. Heat up a pan over medium heat, add beef, stir and brown for 10 minutes.

3. Add chili powder mix, stir, take off heat and stuff pepper halves with this mix.

4. Sprinkle cheese all over, place peppers in your air fryer's basket and cook them at 350 degrees F for 6 minutes.

5. Arrange peppers on a platter and serve them with sour cream on the side.

Enjoy!

Nutrition: calories 170, fat 22, fiber 3, carbs 6, protein 27

Cheesy Zucchini Snack

Preparation time: 10 minutes **Cooking time:** 8 minutes **Servings:** 4

Ingredients:

- 1 cup mozzarella, shredded
- ¼ cup tomato sauce
- 1 zucchini, sliced
- Salt and black pepper to the taste
- A pinch of cumin
- Cooking spray

Directions:

1. Arrange zucchini slices in your air fryer's basket, spray them with cooking oil, spread tomato sauce all over, them, season with salt, pepper, cumin, sprinkle mozzarella at the end and cook them at 320 degrees F for 8 minutes.
2. Arrange them on a platter and serve as a snack.

Enjoy!

Nutrition: calories 150, fat 4, fiber 2, carbs 12, protein 4

Spinach Balls

Preparation time: 10 minutes **Cooking time:** 7 minutes **Servings:** 30

Ingredients:

- 4 tablespoons butter, melted
- 2 eggs
- 1 cup flour
- 16 ounces spinach
- 1/3 cup feta cheese, crumbled
- ¼ teaspoon nutmeg, ground
- 1/3 cup parmesan, grated
- Salt and black pepper to the taste
- 1 tablespoon onion powder
- 3 tablespoons whipping cream
- 1 teaspoon garlic powder

Directions:

1. In your blender, mix spinach with butter, eggs, flour, feta cheese, parmesan, nutmeg, whipping cream, salt, pepper, onion and garlic pepper, blend very well and keep in the freezer for 10 minutes.

2. Shape 30 spinach balls, place them in your air fryer's basket and cook at 300 degrees F for 7 minutes.
3. Serve as a party appetizer.

Enjoy!

Nutrition: calories 60, fat 5, fiber 1, carbs 1, protein 2

Mushrooms Appetizer

Preparation time: 10 minutes **Cooking time:** 10 minutes
Servings: 4

Ingredients:

- ¼ cup mayonnaise
- 1 teaspoon garlic powder
- 1 small yellow onion, chopped
- 24 ounces white mushroom caps
- Salt and black pepper to the taste
- 1 teaspoon curry powder
- 4 ounces cream cheese, soft
- ¼ cup sour cream
- ½ cup Mexican cheese, shredded
- 1 cup shrimp, cooked, peeled, deveined and chopped

Directions:

1. In a bowl, mix mayo with garlic powder, onion, curry powder, cream cheese, sour cream, Mexican cheese, shrimp, salt and pepper to the taste and whisk well.

2. Stuff mushrooms with this mix, place them in your air fryer's basket and cook at 300 degrees F for 10 minutes.

3. Arrange on a platter and serve as an appetizer.

Enjoy!

Nutrition: calories 200, fat 20, fiber 3, carbs 16, protein 14

Cheesy Party Wings

Preparation time: 10 minutes **Cooking time:** 12 minutes
Servings: 6

Ingredients:

- 6 pound chicken wings, halved
- Salt and black pepper to the taste
- ½ teaspoon Italian seasoning
- 2 tablespoons butter
- ½ cup parmesan cheese, grated
- A pinch of red pepper flakes, crushed
- 1 teaspoon garlic powder
- 1 egg

Directions:

1. Arrange chicken wings in your air fryer's basket and cook at 390 degrees F and cook for 9 minutes.
2. Meanwhile, in your blender, mix butter with cheese, egg, salt, pepper, pepper flakes, garlic powder and Italian seasoning and blend very well.

3. Take chicken wings out, pour cheese sauce over them, toss to coat well and cook in your air fryer's basket at 390 degrees F for 3 minutes.

4. Serve them as an appetizer.

Enjoy!

Nutrition: calories 204, fat 8, fiber 1, carbs 18, protein 14

Cheese Sticks

Preparation time: 1 hour and 10 minutes **Cooking time:** 8 minutes **Servings:** 16

Ingredients:

- 2 eggs, whisked
- Salt and black pepper to the taste
- 8 mozzarella cheese strings, cut into halves
- 1 cup parmesan, grated
- 1 tablespoon Italian seasoning
- Cooking spray
- 1 garlic clove, minced

Directions:

1. In a bowl, mix parmesan with salt, pepper, Italian seasoning and garlic and stir well.
2. Put whisked eggs in another bowl.
3. Dip mozzarella sticks in egg mixture, then in cheese mix.
4. Dip them again in egg and in parmesan mix and keep them in the freezer for 1 hour.

5. Spray cheese sticks with cooking oil, place them in your air fryer's basket and cook at 390 degrees F for 8 minutes flipping them halfway.

6. Arrange them on a platter and serve as an appetizer.

Enjoy!

Nutrition: calories 140, fat 5, fiber 1, carbs 3, protein 4

Sweet Bacon Snack

Preparation time: 10 minutes **Cooking time:** 30 minutes
Servings: 16

Ingredients:

- ½ teaspoon cinnamon powder
- 16 bacon slices
- 1 tablespoon avocado oil
- 3 ounces dark chocolate
- 1 teaspoon maple extract

Directions:

1. Arrange bacon slices in your air fryer's basket, sprinkle cinnamon mix over them and cook them at 300 degrees F for 30 minutes.
2. Heat up a pot with the oil over medium heat, add chocolate and stir until it melts.
3. Add maple extract, stir, take off heat and leave aside to cool down a bit.
4. Take bacon strips out of the oven, leave them to cool down, dip each in chocolate mix, place them on a

parchment paper and leave them to cool down completely.

5. Serve cold as a snack.

Enjoy!

Nutrition: calories 200, fat 4, fiber 5, carbs 12, protein 3

Chicken Rolls

Preparation time: 2 hours and 10 minutes **Cooking time:** 10 minutes **Servings:** 12

Ingredients:

- 4 ounces blue cheese, crumbled
- 2 cups chicken, cooked and chopped
- Salt and black pepper to the taste
- 2 green onions, chopped
- 2 celery stalks, finely chopped
- ½ cup tomato sauce
- 12 egg roll wrappers
- Cooking spray

Directions:

1. In a bowl, mix chicken meat with blue cheese, salt, pepper, green onions, celery and tomato sauce, stir well and keep in the fridge for 2 hours.
2. Place egg wrappers on a working surface, divide chicken mix on them, roll and seal edges.

3. Place rolls in your air fryer's basket, spray them with cooking oil and cook at 350 degrees F for 10 minutes, flipping them halfway.

Enjoy!

Nutrition: calories 220, fat 7, fiber 2, carbs 14, protein 10

Tasty Kale and Celery Crackers

Preparation time: 10 minutes **Cooking time:** 20 minutes
Servings: 6

Ingredients:

- 2 cups flax seed, ground
- 2 cups flax seed, soaked overnight and drained
- 4 bunches kale, chopped
- 1 bunch basil, chopped
- ½ bunch celery, chopped
- 4 garlic cloves, minced
- 1/3 cup olive oil

Directions:

1. In your food processor mix ground flaxseed with celery, kale, basil and garlic and blend well.
2. Add oil and soaked flaxseed and blend again, spread in your air fryer's pan, cut into medium crackers and cook them at 380 degrees F for 20 minutes.
3. Divide into bowls and serve as an appetizer.

Enjoy!

Nutrition: calories 143, fat 1, fiber 2, carbs 8, protein 4

Egg White Chips

Preparation time: 5 minutes **Cooking time:** 8 minutes **Servings:** 2

Ingredients:

- ½ tablespoon water
- 2 tablespoons parmesan, shredded
- 4 eggs whites
- Salt and black pepper to the taste

Directions:

1. In a bowl, mix egg whites with salt, pepper and water and whisk well.
2. Spoon this into a muffin pan that fits your air fryer, sprinkle cheese on top, introduce in your air fryer and cook at 350 degrees F for 8 minutes.
3. Arrange egg white chips on a platter and serve as a snack.

Enjoy!

Nutrition: calories 180, fat 2, fiber 1, carbs 12, protein 7

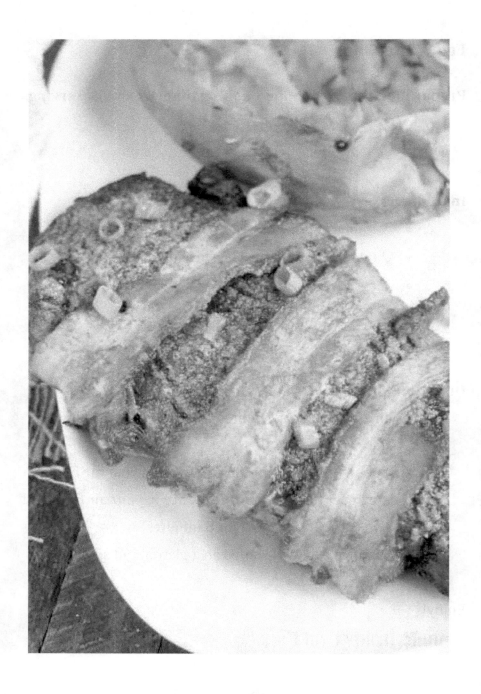

Tuna Cakes

Preparation time: 10 minutes **Cooking time:** 10 minutes
Servings: 12

Ingredients:

- 15 ounces canned tuna, drain and flaked
- 3 eggs
- ½ teaspoon dill, dried
- 1 teaspoon parsley, dried
- ½ cup red onion, chopped
- 1 teaspoon garlic powder
- Salt and black pepper to the taste
- Cooking spray

Directions:

1. In a bowl, mix tuna with salt, pepper, dill, parsley, onion, garlic powder and eggs, stir well and shape medium cakes out of this mix.
2. Place tuna cakes in your air fryer's basket, spray them with cooking oil and cook at 350 degrees F for 10 minutes, flipping them halfway.
3. Arrange them on a platter and serve as an appetizer.

Enjoy!

Nutrition: calories 140, fat 2, fiber 1, carbs 8, protein 6

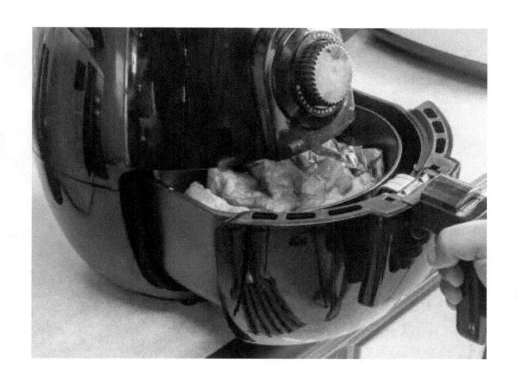

Calamari and Shrimp Snack

Preparation time: 10 minutes **Cooking time:** 20 minutes

Servings: 1

Ingredients:

- 8 ounces calamari, cut into medium rings
- 7 ounces shrimp, peeled and deveined
- 1 eggs
- 3 tablespoons white flour
- 1 tablespoon olive oil
- 2 tablespoons avocado, chopped
- 1 teaspoon tomato paste
- 1 tablespoon mayonnaise
- A splash of Worcestershire sauce
- 1 teaspoon lemon juice
- Salt and black pepper to the taste
- ½ teaspoon turmeric powder

Directions:

1. In a bowl, whisk egg with oil, add calamari rings and shrimp and toss to coat.

2. In another bowl, mix flour with salt, pepper and turmeric and stir.
3. Dredge calamari and shrimp in this mix, place them in your air fryer's basket and cook at 350 degrees F for 9 minutes, flipping them once.
4. Meanwhile, in a bowl, mix avocado with mayo and tomato paste and mash using a fork.
5. Add Worcestershire sauce, lemon juice, salt and pepper and stir well.
6. Arrange calamari and shrimp on a platter and serve with the sauce on the side.

Enjoy!

Nutrition: calories 288, fat 23, fiber 3, carbs 10, protein 15

Cauliflower Cakes

Preparation time: 10 minutes **Cooking time:** 10 minutes

Servings: 6

Ingredients:

- 3 and ½ cups cauliflower rice
- 2 eggs
- ¼ cup white flour
- ½ cup parmesan, grated
- Salt and black pepper to the taste
- Cooking spray

Directions:

1. In a bowl, mix cauliflower rice with salt and pepper, stir and squeeze excess water.
2. Transfer cauliflower to another bowl, add eggs, salt, pepper, flour and parmesan, stir really well and shape your cakes.
3. Grease your air fryer with cooking spray, heat it up at 400 degrees, add cauliflower cakes and cook them for 10 minutes flipping them halfway.
4. Divide cakes on plates and serve as a side dish.

Enjoy!

Nutrition: calories 125, fat 2, fiber 6, carbs 8, protein 3

Creamy Brussels Sprouts

Preparation time: 10 minutes **Cooking time:** 25 minutes

Servings: 8

Ingredients:

- 3 pounds Brussels sprouts, halved
- A drizzle of olive oil
- 1 pound bacon, chopped
- Salt and black pepper to the taste
- 4 tablespoons butter
- 3 shallots, chopped
- 1 cup milk
- 2 cups heavy cream
- ¼ teaspoon nutmeg, ground
- 3 tablespoons prepared horseradish

Directions:

1. Preheated you air fryer at 370 degrees F, add oil, bacon, salt and pepper and Brussels sprouts and toss.
2. Add butter, shallots, heavy cream, milk, nutmeg and horseradish, toss again and cook for 25 minutes.
3. Divide among plates and serve as a side dish.

Enjoy!

Nutrition: calories 214, fat 5, fiber 8, carbs 12, protein 5

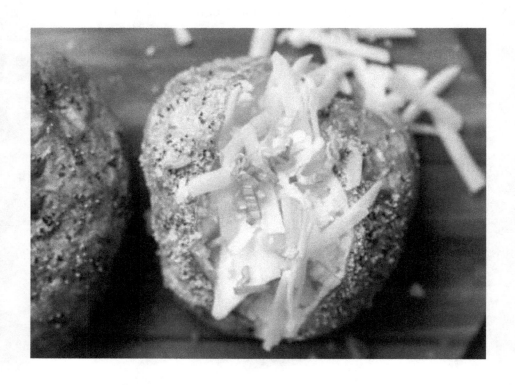

Cheddar Biscuits

Preparation time: 10 minutes **Cooking time:** 20 minutes
Servings: 8

Ingredients:

- 2 and 1/3 cup self-rising flour
- ½ cup butter+ 1 tablespoon, melted
- 2 tablespoons sugar
- ½ cup cheddar cheese, grated
- 1 and 1/3 cup buttermilk
- 1 cup flour

Directions:

1. In a bowl, mix self-rising flour with ½ cup butter, sugar, cheddar cheese and buttermilk and stir until you obtain a dough.
2. Spread 1 cup flour on a working surface, roll dough, flatten it, cut 8 circles with a cookie cutter and coat them with flour.
3. Line your air fryer's basket with tin foil, add biscuits, brush them with melted butter and cook them at 380 degrees F for 20 minutes.
4. Divide among plates and serve as a side.

Enjoy!

Nutrition: calories 221, fat 3, fiber 8, carbs 12, protein 4

Zucchini Fries

Preparation time: 10 minutes **Cooking time:** 12 minutes

Servings: 4

Ingredients:

- 1 zucchini, cut into medium sticks
- A drizzle of olive oil
- Salt and black pepper to the taste
- 2 eggs, whisked
- 1 cup bread crumbs
- ½ cup flour

Directions:

1. Put flour in a bowl and mix with salt and pepper and stir.
2. Put breadcrumbs in another bowl.
3. In a third bowl mix eggs with a pinch of salt and pepper.
4. Dredge zucchini fries in flour, then in eggs and in bread crumbs at the end.

5. Grease your air fryer with some olive oil, heat up at 400 degrees F, add zucchini fries and cook them for 12 minutes.

6. Serve them as a side dish.

Enjoy!

Nutrition: calories 172, fat 3, fiber 3, carbs 7, protein 3

Delicious Red Snapper

Preparation time: 30 minutes **Cooking time:** 15 minutes
Servings: 4

Ingredients:

- 1 big red snapper, cleaned and scored
- Salt and black pepper to the taste
- 3 garlic cloves, minced
- 1 jalapeno, chopped
- ¼ pound okra, chopped
- 1 tablespoon butter
- 2 tablespoons olive oil
- 1 red bell pepper, chopped
- 2 tablespoons white wine
- 2 tablespoons parsley, chopped

Directions:

1. In a bowl, mix jalapeno, wine with garlic, stir well and rub snapper with this mix.
2. Season fish with salt and pepper and leave it aside for 30 minutes.

3. Meanwhile, heat up a pan with 1 tablespoon butter over medium heat, add bell pepper and okra, stir and cook for 5 minutes.

4. Stuff red snapper's belly with this mix, also add parsley and rub with the olive oil.

5. Place in preheated air fryer and cook at 400 degrees F for 15 minutes, flipping the fish halfway.

6. Divide among plates and serve.

Enjoy!

Nutrition: calories 261, fat 7, fiber 18, carbs 28, protein 18

Snapper Fillets and Veggies

Preparation time: 10 minutes **Cooking time:** 14 minutes
Servings: 2

Ingredients:

- 2 red snapper fillets, boneless
- 1 tablespoon olive oil
- ½ cup red bell pepper, chopped
- ½ cup green bell pepper, chopped
- ½ cup leeks, chopped
- Salt and black pepper to the taste
- 1 teaspoon tarragon, dried
- A splash of white wine

Directions:

1. In a heat proof dish that fits your air fryer, mix fish fillets with salt, pepper, oil, green bell pepper, red bell pepper, leeks, tarragon and wine, toss well everything, introduce in preheated air fryer at 350 degrees F and cook for 14 minutes, flipping fish fillets halfway.
2. Divide fish and veggies on plates and serve warm.

Enjoy!

Nutrition: calories 300, fat 12, fiber 8, carbs 29, protein 12

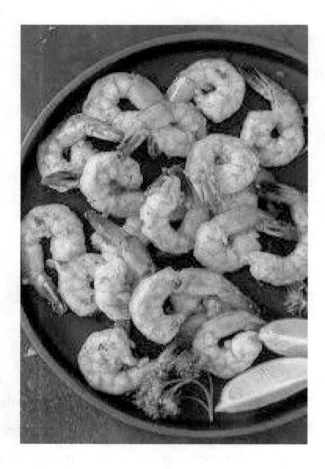

Air Fried Branzino

Preparation time: 10 minutes **Cooking time:** 10 minutes
Servings: 4

Ingredients:

- Zest from 1 lemon, grated
- Zest from 1 orange, grated
- Juice from ½ lemon
- Juice from ½ orange
- Salt and black pepper to the taste
- 4 medium branzino fillets, boneless
- ½ cup parsley, chopped
- 2 tablespoons olive oil
- A pinch of red pepper flakes, crushed

Directions:

1. In a large bowl, mix fish fillets with lemon zest, orange zest, lemon juice, orange juice, salt, pepper, oil and pepper flakes, toss really well, transfer fillets to your preheated air fryer at 350 degrees F and bake for 10 minutes, flipping fillets once.

2. Divide fish on plates, sprinkle with parsley and serve right away.

Enjoy!

Nutrition: calories 261, fat 8, fiber 12, carbs 21, protein 12

Lemon Sole and Swiss Chard

Preparation time: 10 minutes **Cooking time:** 14 minutes
Servings: 4

Ingredients:

- 1 teaspoon lemon zest, grated
- 4 white bread slices, quartered
- ¼ cup walnuts, chopped
- ¼ cup parmesan, grated
- 4 tablespoons olive oil
- 4 sole fillets, boneless
- Salt and black pepper to the taste
- 4 tablespoons butter
- ¼ cup lemon juice
- 3 tablespoons capers
- 2 garlic cloves, minced
- 2 bunches Swiss chard, chopped

Directions:

1. In your food processor, mix bread with walnuts, cheese and lemon zest and pulse well.

2. Add half of the olive oil, pulse really well again and leave aside for now.
3. Heat up a pan with the butter over medium heat, add lemon juice, salt, pepper and capers, stir well, add fish and toss it.
4. Transfer fish to your preheated air fryer's basket, top with bread mix you've made at the beginning and cook at 350 degrees F for 14 minutes.
5. Meanwhile, heat up another pan with the rest of the oil, add garlic, Swiss chard, salt and pepper, stir gently, cook for 2 minutes and take off heat.
6. Divide fish on plates and serve with sautéed chard on the side.

Enjoy!

Nutrition: calories 321, fat 7, fiber 18, carbs 27, protein 12

Salmon and Blackberry Glaze

Preparation time: 10 minutes **Cooking time:** 33 minutes
Servings: 4

Ingredients:

- 1 cup water
- 1 inch ginger piece, grated
- Juice from ½ lemon
- 12 ounces blackberries
- 1 tablespoon olive oil
- ¼ cup sugar
- 4 medium salmon fillets, skinless
- Salt and black pepper to the taste

Directions:

1. Heat up a pot with the water over medium high heat, add ginger, lemon juice and blackberries, stir, bring to a boil, cook for 4-5 minutes, take off heat, strain into a bowl, return to pan and combine with sugar.
2. Stir this mix, bring to a simmer over medium low heat and cook for 20 minutes.

3. Leave blackberry sauce to cool down, brush salmon with it, season with salt and pepper, drizzle olive oil all over and rub fish well.
4. Place fish in your preheated air fryer at 350 degrees F and cook for 10 minutes, flipping fish fillets once.
5. Divide among plates, drizzle some of the remaining blackberry sauce all over and serve.

Enjoy!

Nutrition: calories 312, fat 4, fiber 9, carbs 19, protein 14

Oriental Fish

Preparation time: 10 minutes **Cooking time:** 12 minutes
Servings: 4

Ingredients:

- 2 pounds red snapper fillets, boneless
- Salt and black pepper to the taste
- 3 garlic cloves, minced
- 1 yellow onion, chopped
- 1 tablespoon tamarind paste
- 1 tablespoon oriental sesame oil
- 1 tablespoon ginger, grated
- 2 tablespoons water
- ½ teaspoon cumin, ground
- 1 tablespoon lemon juice
- 3 tablespoons mint, chopped

Directions:

1. In your food processor, mix garlic with onion, salt, pepper, tamarind paste, sesame oil, ginger, water and cumin, pulse well and rub fish with this mix.

2. Place fish in your preheated air fryer at 320 degrees F and cook for 12 minutes, flipping fish halfway.
3. Divide fish on plates, drizzle lemon juice all over, sprinkle mint and serve right away.

Enjoy!

Nutrition: calories 241, fat 8, fiber 16, carbs 17, protein 12

Delicious French Cod

Preparation time: 10 minutes **Cooking time:** 22 minutes

Servings: 4

Ingredients:

- 2 tablespoons olive oil
- 1 yellow onion, chopped
- ½ cup white wine
- 2 garlic cloves, minced
- 14 ounces canned tomatoes, stewed
- 3 tablespoons parsley, chopped
- 2 pounds cod, boneless
- Salt and black pepper to the taste
- 2 tablespoons butter

Directions:

1. Heat up a pan with the oil over medium heat, add garlic and onion, stir and cook for 5 minutes.
2. Add wine, stir and cook for 1 minute more.
3. Add tomatoes, stir, bring to a boil, cook for 2 minutes, add parsley, stir again and take off heat.

4. Pour this mix into a heat proof dish that fits your air fryer, add fish, season it with salt and pepper and cook in your fryer at 350 degrees F for 14 minutes.
5. Divide fish and tomatoes mix on plates and serve.

Enjoy!

Nutrition: calories 231, fat 8, fiber 12, carbs 26, protein 14